FLOW

A Clearer Way to Understand and Protect Your Heart

NACHIKET J. PATEL, MD, FACC, FSCAI
Interventional Cardiologist · Flow Heart & Vascular

FLOWPRESS
Tempe, Arizona

FlowPress
Tempe, Arizona, USA

ISBN (Hardcover): 979-8-9941203-1-6
ISBN (Paperback): 979-8-9941203-0-9
ISBN (eBook): 979-8-9941203-2-3

For permission requests: info@flowheartandvascular.com
flowheartandvascular.com
First Edition, 2026

To my patients, who have trusted me in their most vulnerable moments: your courage, your questions, and your stories are the heartbeat of my work.

And to anyone who has waited in a hospital hallway, unsure what comes next: this book is for you.
You deserve clarity. You deserve hope.

Where Flow falters, disease begins.

Where Flow is understood, fear fades.

Where Flow is restored, the future changes.

About the Author

Nachiket J. Patel, MD, FACC, FSCAI, is an interventional cardiologist and founder of Flow Heart & Vascular, cardiovascular practice in Mesa, Arizona.

He is board-certified in cardiovascular disease and interventional cardiology and serves as a Clinical Assistant Professor of Medicine at the University of Arizona College of Medicine – Phoenix. His academic work includes peer-reviewed publications and clinical research in cardiovascular medicine.

Dr. Patel has spent thousands of hours working inside coronary and peripheral arteries during some of the most critical moments in patients' lives. That vantage point shapes how he practices and teaches. A visible blockage is only one part of the story; biology, blood flow, symptoms, and time give a finding its meaning and guide what should happen next.

Whether caring for a patient, teaching, or explaining new research, Dr. Patel returns to three practical questions: What is happening? What can a test show, and what can it not show? What should happen next?

He wrote *Flow: A Clearer Way to Understand and Protect Your Heart* to bring that conversation to readers before uncertainty becomes confusion, a decision feels rushed, or an opportunity to act is missed.

Dr. Patel lives and practices in Arizona. Outside of medicine, he enjoys hiking Arizona's desert trails and spending time with his family.

flowheartandvascular.com

A Note to Readers

This book provides general education. It cannot diagnose a condition, replace personalized medical advice, or account for every detail of your health. Medical knowledge changes, and recommendations may change with it. The evidence for this edition was reviewed through July 2026. Use the book to understand a conversation and ask better questions, not to change treatment on your own.

If you think you may be having an emergency, call 911 or your local emergency service. Do not use this book, a worksheet, a wearable, or a prior test result to decide that a new or severe symptom is safe.

The patient stories are composites. Identifying details, including age, sex, medical history, and circumstances, have been altered or combined to protect privacy. These stories illustrate real patterns of cardiovascular care, not identifiable individuals.

The figures simplify complex anatomy and biology so the main idea is easier to understand. They are teaching illustrations, not personalized images of any reader's heart or arteries.

USE THIS BOOK TO ASK BETTER QUESTIONS
IT IS A GUIDE TO UNDERSTANDING AND SHARED DECISIONS, NOT A SET OF INSTRUCTIONS FOR CHANGING CARE ON YOUR OWN.

Start Here: When Symptoms May Be an Emergency

Call 911 now if you have any of the following:

- New chest pressure, heaviness, squeezing, or tightness that is happening now, is severe or worsening, lasts more than a few minutes, repeatedly returns, or occurs at rest or with minimal exertion.
- Chest discomfort with breathlessness, sweating, nausea, fainting, marked weakness, or discomfort spreading to the arm, jaw, neck, back, or shoulder.
- Sudden severe breathlessness; fainting; signs of stroke such as facial droop, arm weakness, or trouble speaking; or any symptom that feels life-threatening.

DO NOT DRIVE YOURSELF

Call 911 and follow the dispatcher's instructions.

If someone collapses, is unresponsive, and is not breathing normally, call 911, begin cardiopulmonary resuscitation (CPR) with chest compressions, and use an automated external defibrillator (AED) as soon as one is available.

Contents

CONTENTS · CONTINUED

Introduction · Why This Book Exists

Most people do not begin thinking seriously about their heart by choice. It usually starts with an unexpected test result, a friend's heart attack, symptoms no one has fully explained, or the silence before a clinician says, "We need to talk."

A plaque-related heart attack may arrive without warning, but it rarely arrives without a history.

Not long ago, a patient sat across from me after a reassuring evaluation. Nothing in front of us called for an urgent procedure.

"I don't feel sick," he said. "But I don't feel safe either."

He was not asking for certainty. He was asking for a way to understand what the test had answered, what it had not, and what should happen next.

With that uncertainty comes a new vocabulary: plaque, ischemia, calcium score, ejection fraction, atrial fibrillation, stent. Each term has a precise clinical meaning, but patients are often asked to assemble the whole picture while worried, tired, or facing a decision they never expected. They are listening, but the story is being told in pieces.

A reassuring test can sound like a universal all-clear. A dramatic image can make a procedure feel inevitable. A symptom can be dismissed because it does not fit the expected pattern. A medicine can seem optional because its benefit is quiet and nothing feels different after the first dose.

I wrote this book to connect those pieces. Years in the catheterization laboratory have shown me how quickly cardiovascular disease can become an emergency. Those same years have shown me the longer story that comes before and after it.

Plaque can develop silently within an artery wall. Blood flow can fail to meet demand. A test can answer one question but not another, and a family can go home with a list of medicines without a clear sense of what happens next.

Flow is the teaching framework I use to keep anatomy, blood flow, symptoms, risk, and the goal of treatment in the same conversation. It treats the arteries as living tissue rather than passive plumbing. Rather than focusing only on visible blockages, it also considers what is happening within the artery wall, whether enough blood is reaching the heart muscle, how hard the heart is working, and how the problem is affecting the person's life.

Flow gives you a practical way to work with uncertainty: recognize urgency, understand the question a test answered, know what a treatment is meant to accomplish, and leave with a clear next step and a time to review it. You do not need medical training to begin.

To understand that longer story, we begin where it can become urgent in minutes: the cath lab.

The goal is not certainty. It is a clearer question, a safer decision, and a next step you understand.

How to Use This Book

You can read this book straight through, but you do not have to. Begin with the question in front of you, then follow the chapters that matter most. The chapters build on one another, but each can stand on its own.

The book focuses mainly on coronary artery disease: plaque, blood flow, symptoms, tests, medicines, and procedures. It also addresses atrial fibrillation, obstructive sleep apnea, heart failure, and recovery where those problems shape real decisions. It is not a comprehensive guide to every heart or vascular condition.

If a symptom may be an emergency, stop here and use the Start Here page before the Contents. Do not use a chapter, worksheet, wearable, or old test result to decide that a new severe symptom is safe.

Find Your Starting Point

YOUR QUESTION	WHERE TO BEGIN
I just had a heart attack, stent, or bypass.	Start with Chapter 15; then use Chapters 13, 14, 16, and 17.
A calcium score or CT scan showed plaque, but I feel well.	Start with Chapter 2; then use Chapters 4, 6, 10, 12, and 14.
I still have symptoms after a reassuring test.	Start with Chapter 10; then read Chapters 8, 11, and 12.
A watch or monitor showed possible atrial fibrillation (AFib), or I have palpitations.	Start with Chapter 9.

YOUR QUESTION	WHERE TO BEGIN
I snore, wake unrefreshed, or have difficult-to-control blood pressure.	Start with Chapter 7.
I am deciding about a test, catheterization, stent, or bypass.	Start with Chapter 12; then read Chapters 13 and 14.
I want to know what I should eat.	Use the Practical Flow Guide in the Toolkit, plus Chapter 4.
I want to understand prevention or inherited risk.	Start with Chapter 4; then read Chapters 6, 7, and 17.
I was told I have heart failure.	Start with Chapter 8; then use Chapters 14–16 with your heart-failure team's plan.
I am helping a family member.	Use the emergency page first if needed; then choose the chapter that matches the immediate question and use the Flow Toolkit to organize the visit.

What Each Part Does

The book moves from story to biology, interpretation, intervention, and action.

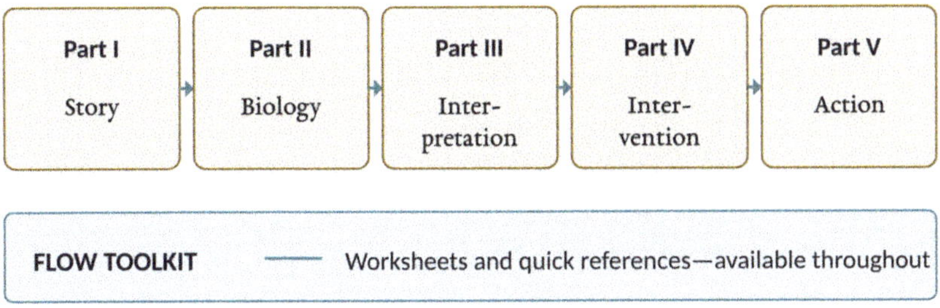

Recurring Guideposts

Flow Takeaway. The central lesson to remember at the end of each chapter.

Flow Truth. A concise principle that clears up a common misconception or sharpens a decision.

Evidence Snapshot / Evidence in Context. Optional research detail showing what a study found, what it means, and what it could not prove.

Safety. Situations that require prompt action or direct instructions from a clinician.

Use the Toolkit When You Need It

The Flow Toolkit is designed for real appointments and real decisions. Use Which Flow Tool Do I Need? to find the worksheet that matches your situation. Read for understanding, not memorization. The goal is to know what the decision means and what should happen next.

PART I

The Disease Behind the Emergency

STORY

A sudden emergency unfolds in minutes. The biology behind it has often been developing for years.

CHAPTER 1

The Day Everything Changes

Even after years in the cath lab, I am still unsettled by how quickly a person can go from talking to having no pulse.

Inside the Cath Lab

A man in his sixties is rushed from the emergency department to the cardiac catheterization laboratory, often called the cath lab. Here, contrast dye and moving X-ray images let us see the heart's arteries and guide treatment. He is sweating but still talking, still hoping this is nothing.

Then the monitor alarms. His heartbeat breaks into a dangerous rhythm. He loses consciousness, and we can no longer feel a pulse. Chest compressions begin, and the room moves at once.

As contrast dye enters an artery supplying his heart, the artery's outline appears on the monitor. We can see where blood flow has stopped. I work to reopen the artery while the rest of the team keeps blood and oxygen moving to his brain and body.

What happened in that room took minutes. What led to it took years.

Two Emergencies in One Room

The patient in the cath lab was living through two related emergencies at once. A heart attack occurs when inadequate blood flow and oxygen injure part of the heart muscle. Cardiac arrest means the heart suddenly stops pumping blood effectively, often because of a dangerous electrical rhythm. A heart attack can trigger cardiac arrest, but most do not, and cardiac arrest can have other causes.

The heart is a muscle, and like every other muscle, it needs oxygen. The coronary arteries arise from the aorta, the body's main artery, and travel across the heart's surface, delivering oxygen-rich blood to the heart muscle. Figure 1.1 shows the major branches: the right coronary artery and the left main coronary artery, which usually divides into the left anterior descending and circumflex arteries.

If blood flow through one suddenly becomes severely reduced or blocked, the heart keeps working while the muscle beyond that point is deprived of oxygen. If flow is not restored quickly, that muscle can be injured.

FLOW TRUTH

A heart attack is a circulation emergency. Cardiac arrest is a pumping emergency. One can trigger the other, but they are not the same.

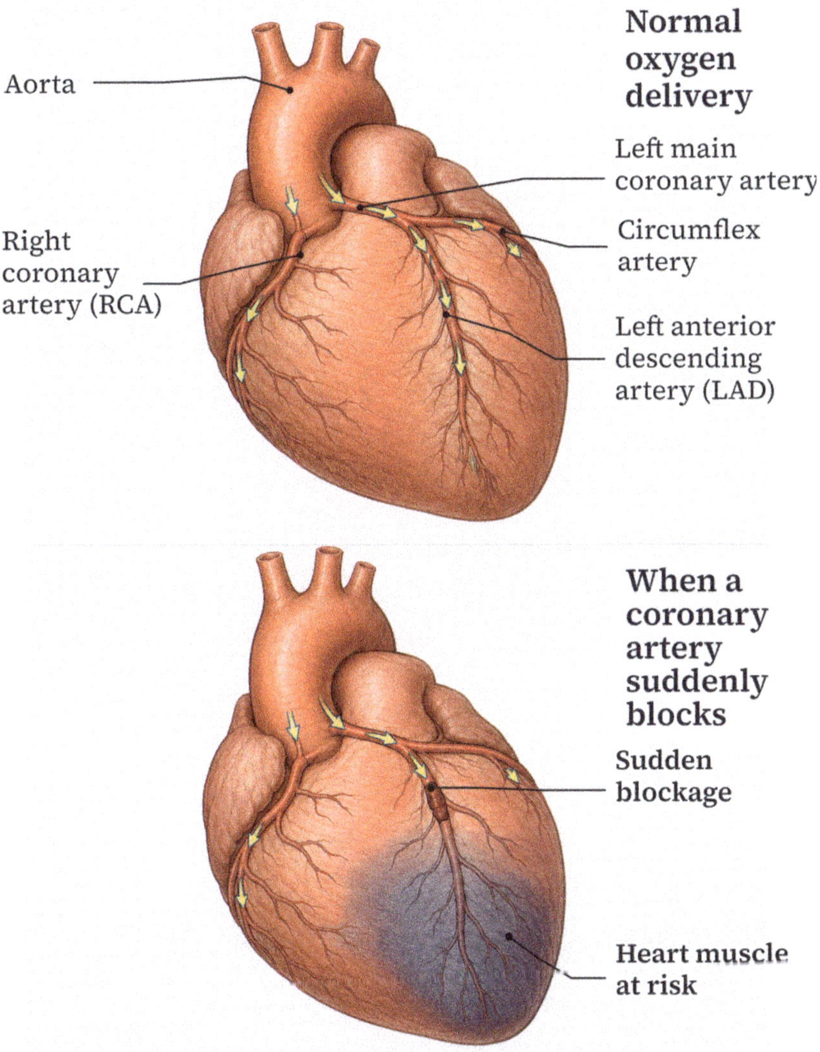

Figure 1.1 · How the Coronary Arteries Feed the Heart. The coronary arteries carry oxygen-rich blood across the heart's surface; a sudden blockage threatens the muscle downstream.

The Slow Biology Behind a "Sudden" Heart Attack

People often say, "He was fine yesterday. Then, out of nowhere, he had a heart attack."

The statement captures the shock of the moment, but it leaves out the years that came before it.

The change can happen in minutes, so it feels as though the disease began that day. Usually, it did not. In many plaque-related heart attacks, the artery wall had been changing quietly for years. Plaque-related coronary disease runs on two clocks: one slow, the other dangerously fast.

I think of arteries as having a kind of memory. Over time, they reflect what they have been exposed to: years of elevated blood pressure, cholesterol-carrying particles entering the artery wall, tobacco, diabetes, disrupted sleep, inherited risk, and the conditions in which a person lives.

Much of that process is silent. There is no alarm when plaque first begins to grow within the artery wall. In some plaques, the artery expands outward, so the channel for blood still looks fairly open. Some plaques develop a large fatty core beneath a thin protective cap.

Then one day, something gives. The plaque surface breaks open, or its protective lining erodes. The body reacts as though it were sealing a wound, and a blood clot begins to form. In minutes, a slow process can become an emergency.

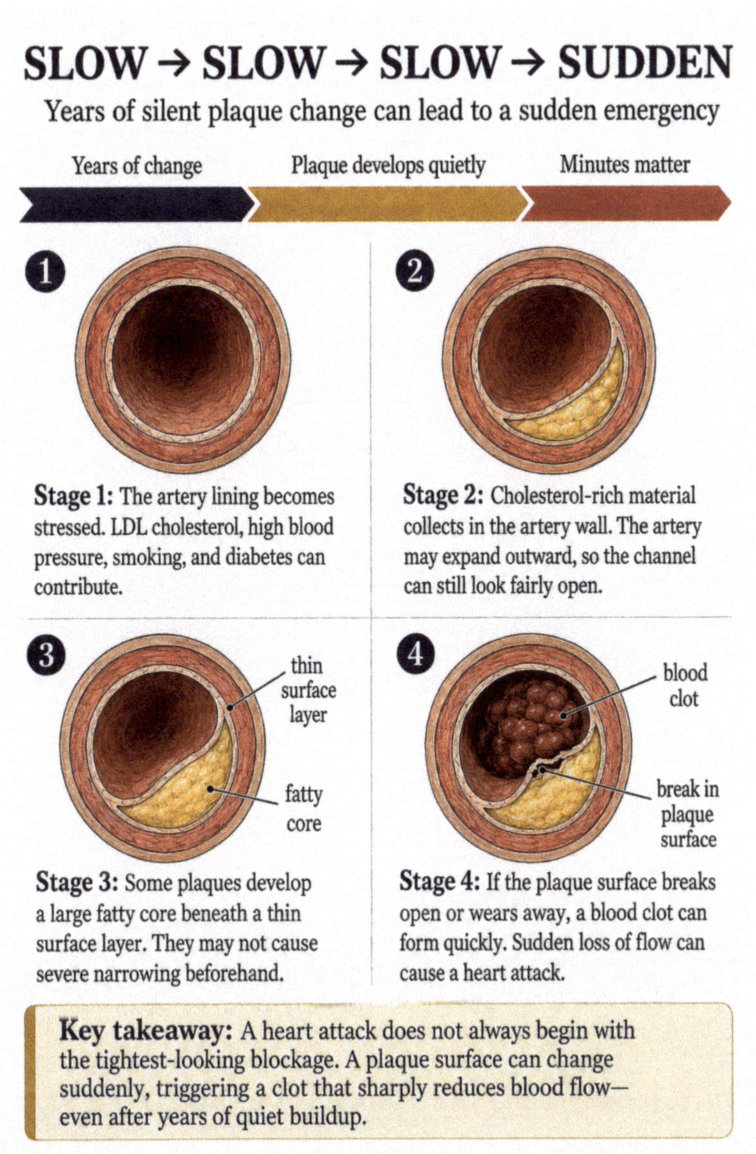

Figure 1.2 · Slow → Slow → Slow → Sudden. The sequence is illustrative, not predictive: it cannot identify which plaque will change or when.

Severe blockages still matter. They can restrict blood flow and cause chest pressure, breathlessness, or reduced exercise tolerance. Whether they need a procedure depends on symptoms, how much they limit blood flow, and the clinical setting. A heart attack can begin at a plaque that had not previously appeared severe, even when another narrowing looked tighter.

The Name for This Pattern: A Type 1 Heart Attack

Doctors call this a type 1 myocardial infarction, or type 1 heart attack. It occurs when a plaque surface ruptures (breaks open) or loses its protective surface through erosion, allowing a clot to form at that site. The clot can sharply reduce or block blood flow within minutes. This book focuses on that plaque-and-clot pattern.

Time Is Muscle. Before Then, Time Is Opportunity.

Once blood flow is suddenly and severely reduced or blocked, every minute puts more heart muscle at risk. That is why cardiologists say, "Time is muscle."

Before an emergency, time is opportunity. Lowering harmful cholesterol and blood pressure, treating diabetes, stopping smoking, becoming more active, and taking medicines shown to help can all lower future risk.

Some measurements improve within weeks; protection from future events builds over months and years. Treatment can be working even when a scan looks unchanged.

The Split-Screen Moment

Many people meet heart disease under fluorescent lights, surrounded by beeping monitors and uncertainty.

I have also sat on the family side of that room.

When my mother needed a procedure on the arteries of her heart, I understood her blockages. I knew the evidence, the expected benefit, and the risks.

That night, my mom, my dad, and I went out to dinner. It was a good night, but afterward, lying in bed, I could not sleep.

I knew her blockages were severe, and I believed the procedure was the right choice. I had explained the risks of that same procedure to thousands of patients: heart attack, stroke, death. I always tell them those complications are uncommon, and that is true. But when the patient is your mother, uncommon is not the same as impossible.

One thought kept circling. The dinner we had just shared might be the last the three of us would ever have.

You don't think like a doctor in those moments.
You think like a son.

Knowing the facts did not make it easier. They made every possibility more vivid.

That is what heart disease can do: split your world in two. One screen holds the clinical data: blood-test results such as troponin, a marker of heart-muscle injury; angiogram images, which use contrast dye to outline the coronary arteries; and ejection fraction, one measure of how well the heart pumps. The other holds everything else: the look on your family members' faces, the conversations you wish you'd had, and the sudden need for more time.

ONE SCREEN

The Data

- Troponin levels
- Angiogram images
- Ejection fraction

THE OTHER SCREEN

Everything Else

- The look on your family's face
- The conversations you wish you'd had
- The sudden need for more time

This book lives in the space between the two screens.

Figure 1.3 · The Split-Screen Moment. One screen holds the clinical data; the other holds everything the data cannot capture.

From the Crisis to the Cause

The crisis is the fast part. Before it, there is time to lower risk; after it, there is still time to protect what comes next. To understand why, we have to look more closely at the living wall of the artery, where plaque can begin long before the channel looks severely narrowed. That is where Chapter 2 begins.

FLOW TAKEAWAY · CHAPTER 1

A plaque-related heart attack may arrive suddenly even though coronary disease has been developing quietly for years. The emergency demands immediate action. Outside an emergency, time is your advantage: use it to identify and treat the risks that allow plaque to grow and become dangerous.

CHAPTER 2

The Endothelium: Your Artery's Protective Lining

You may picture a heart attack like a clogged kitchen sink. Material builds up inside a pipe, the opening grows tighter, and eventually nothing gets through.

That picture explains one part of coronary disease. A severe narrowing can restrict blood flow and cause real symptoms. But it cannot explain every heart attack.

I think of a patient I will return to in Chapter 10. He was in his early fifties, ran regularly, coached his daughter's soccer team, and felt well. Eight months before I met him, a stress test had been reassuring. Then he arrived by ambulance having a heart attack.

His family kept returning to the same question: How could the stress test be normal and this happen months later?

The test had answered an important question. Under the conditions tested, it had found no sign that part of his heart was receiving too little blood. It had not mapped every plaque inside his artery walls or predicted whether one might later change and trigger a clot. The result was reassuring, but the reassurance had limits.

In a case like his, the plaque that later ruptured may have caused only a mild, nonobstructive narrowing, not enough to create the blood-flow problem many stress tests are designed to detect. Studies that looked at arteries before a heart attack found that many sites where the heart attack began had previously narrowed the artery by less than half.

To understand how both facts can be true, we need a better picture of an artery.

Your Arteries Are Not Pipes

The pipe picture is useful when an artery has a severe, fixed narrowing. It becomes incomplete when we imagine the artery as passive plumbing and plaque as debris piling up only in the open channel.

Arteries are living tissue. They widen and tighten, sense pressure and injury, interact with the blood moving through them, and respond to treatment over time. For now, picture two parts: the open channel where blood flows, and the living wall around it. The wall's innermost surface is a layer of cells called the endothelium.

The Artery's One-Cell-Thick Working Surface

The endothelium is only one cell thick, but it is not just a coating. It helps the artery widen when more blood is needed, restrains unnecessary clotting, regulates inflammation and repair, and helps control how cholesterol-carrying particles and immune cells move into the artery wall.

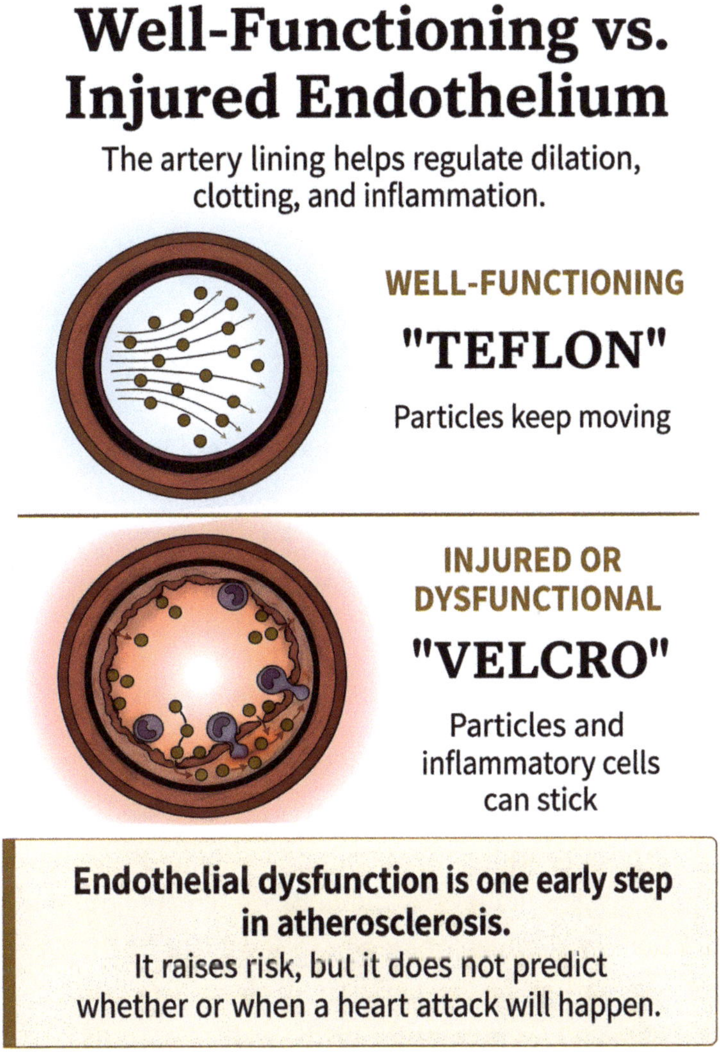

Figure 2.1 · Well-Functioning and Dysfunctional Endothelium: A Teflon-and-Velcro Metaphor. A healthy lining regulates blood flow, inflammation, and clotting. When dysfunctional, it can become more permeable and adhesive, allowing low-density lipoprotein (LDL) particles to enter the wall and inflammatory cells to adhere to the lining and migrate into the wall more readily.

Teflon Versus Velcro

The easiest way to picture the endothelium is to think of a well-functioning surface as Teflon-like. It captures how the lining helps blood move smoothly and keeps the artery's internal environment well regulated.

When the lining is repeatedly injured or stops working normally, it becomes leakier and stickier. LDL is often called the "bad" cholesterol; think L for lousy. More precisely, LDL particles carry cholesterol in the blood, and those particles and inflammatory cells can enter the wall more easily. The change is gradual, not an on-and-off switch, and endothelial function can improve with treatment.

Plaque Grows in the Wall, Not in the Pipe

Plaque does not sit in the open channel like gum stuck inside a pipe. It develops beneath the endothelium, within the artery wall.

When cholesterol-carrying particles enter and remain in the artery wall, the immune system responds. Over time, cholesterol, inflammatory cells, and scar-like tissue can build into plaque. As plaque grows, the wall may expand outward to make room for it. For a time, the artery channel for blood can stay fairly open. A person may feel well, and a stress test may show no reduction in blood flow, even though plaque is present inside the wall.

This slow buildup of plaque in artery walls is called atherosclerosis. When it affects the coronary arteries, it is called coronary atherosclerosis or coronary artery disease.

If the sink image makes plaque seem as though it is piled in the middle of the artery, a pimple offers one useful correction. A pimple develops beneath a surface and can break open suddenly. Plaque is far more complex, but it also grows beneath a lining, inside the artery wall.

Why Similar Narrowings Can Carry Different Risk

Plaques are not all built the same. Some have a thicker protective cap and less fatty or inflamed material. Others contain more plaque within the wall or have a thinner cap over a larger fatty core. Those differences help explain why similar-looking narrowings can carry different risk.

Plaques With Different Risk Features

Risk depends on more than the degree of narrowing.

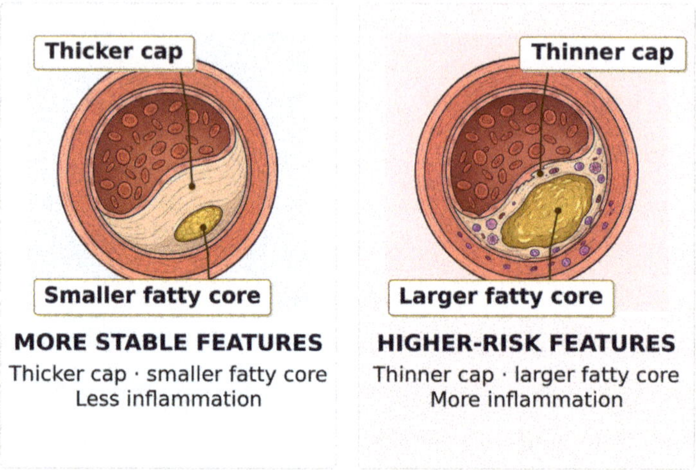

WHAT THE COMPARISON SHOWS

- On an angiogram, plaques with different wall features can look similarly narrowed.
- A thin cap, large fatty core, and more inflammation are associated with greater risk.
- Percent narrowing does not tell the whole story.
- No image can predict with certainty which plaque will cause a future event.

Figure 2.2 · Plaques With Different Risk Features. Similar degrees of narrowing can hide different plaque burdens and biological features. A thinner cap, a larger fatty core, and more inflammation are associated with higher risk, but no image can tell with certainty which plaque will cause trouble.

EVIDENCE SNAPSHOT 2.1

Why a Mild-Looking Narrowing Can Still Matter

PROSPECT · N ENGL J MED, 2011

WHAT WAS STUDIED

After a heart attack or serious heart-related chest pain, researchers used imaging from inside the arteries to study plaques that had not been treated.

WHAT RESEARCHERS FOUND

Later problems sometimes arose from areas that had looked only mildly narrowed on angiography but contained more plaque or a large fatty core beneath a thin cap. Most later events were hospitalizations for worsening chest pain, not heart attacks or sudden death.

WHAT THIS MEANS

The percentage of narrowing is not the whole story; features within the artery wall matter too.

IMPORTANT LIMIT

These patients had already experienced a heart attack or serious heart-related chest pain. The study identified features associated with higher risk but could not reliably predict which individual plaque would later cause trouble.

A mild-looking narrowing can still hide substantial plaque.

THE PICTURE IS ONLY PART OF THE STORY

When a plaque's surface breaks open or loses its protective lining through erosion, a clot may form quickly. That is the sudden step described in Chapter 1.

> **FLOW TRUTH**
>
> A fixed narrowing may limit blood flow, especially when the heart works harder. A heart attack can also begin when the surface of a less severe plaque changes and a clot forms. One question asks how blood flows today. The other asks what could happen later. No single narrowing percentage answers both.

Because we cannot reliably identify which plaque will cause a future event, prevention protects the whole arterial system. A procedure treats a particular narrowing or blockage when doing so is expected to help. Chapter 13 examines an emerging exception under study: preventive percutaneous coronary intervention (PCI), usually a stent procedure, for a narrowly selected high-risk plaque identified with imaging from inside the artery.

What the Stress Test Had Actually Shown

> **MYTH / REALITY**
>
> **MYTH:** A normal stress test means there is no plaque.
>
> **REALITY:** A stress test looks for a blood-flow problem under the conditions tested. It does not map every plaque inside the artery wall.

A reassuring result lowers concern about a major flow-limiting problem at that time. New or worsening symptoms create a new question and deserve reassessment.

The Living Wall Can Respond to Treatment

Because an artery is living tissue, the treatment you begin or continue can change its biology. It can improve lining function, reduce harmful particles reaching the wall, and make plaque less likely to cause trouble.

Later chapters show how blood pressure, cholesterol, diabetes, tobacco, movement, sleep, and medicines shape that biology.

Chapter 3 turns these ideas into three questions you can use to interpret a test and decide what comes next.

> **FLOW PRACTICE · START WITH FIVE MINUTES**
>
> If activity is safe for you, take a five-minute walk or add five minutes of adapted movement today. The point is not intensity. It is beginning a pattern you can repeat.

> **FLOW TAKEAWAY · CHAPTER 2**
>
> An artery is a living wall surrounding an open channel. Plaque can be present without severe narrowing. If you are given a narrowing percentage, ask what plaque burden, blood flow, symptoms, and overall risk add to the picture.

CHAPTER 3

Flow: A Sharper Way to See Heart Disease

Imagine two patients who come to me in the same month. Each angiogram shows a 50 percent narrowing in one coronary artery. The images look alike. The decisions do not.

A percentage feels like an answer. Most of the time, it is only the beginning of one.

The Pipe Picture: Useful, but Incomplete

The pipe model asks where an artery is narrowed. That matters: a tight narrowing can limit blood flow, cause symptoms, and sometimes call for a procedure. But a narrowing percentage is not a diagnosis or a decision by itself.

The Flow Engine

Chapter 2 introduced the endothelium and the artery wall. The Flow framework keeps both in view and adds the microcirculation, the smallest vessels that match blood flow to the heart's needs. Together, they form the Flow Engine, a practical model of the connected biology behind the three Flow questions.

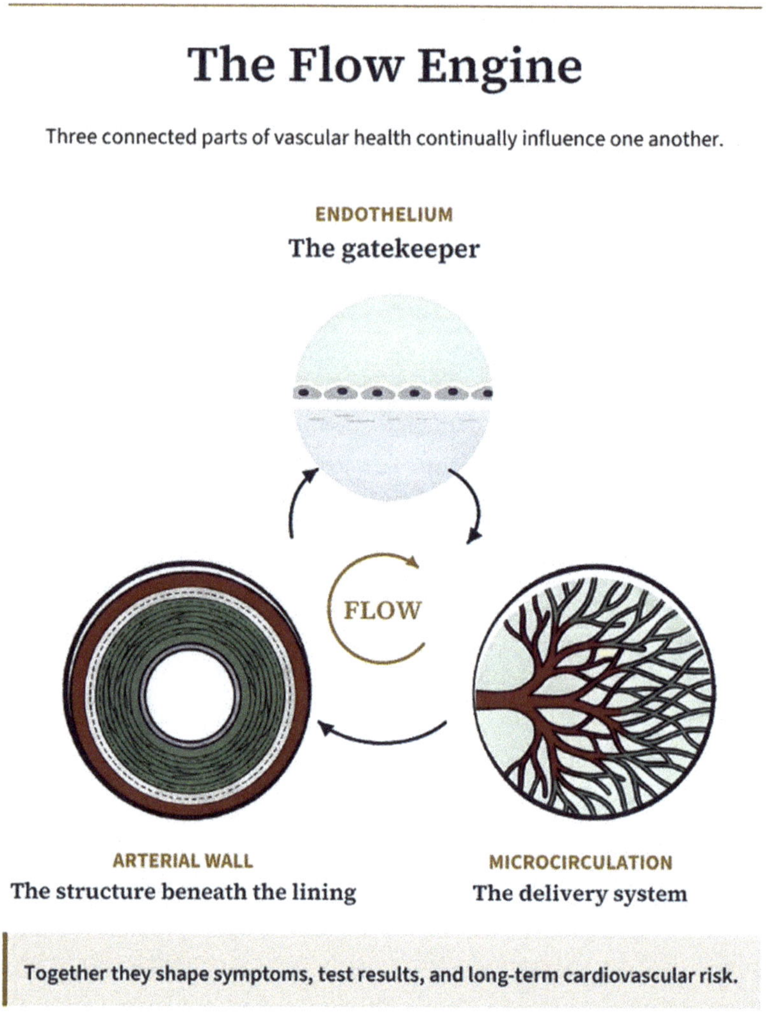

Figure 3.1 · The Flow Engine. The Flow Engine keeps the endothelium, artery wall, and microcirculation in the same view.

The Endothelium: The Gatekeeper

The endothelium is the artery's thin working surface. It senses blood flow, helps the vessel widen, and helps regulate inflammation and clotting.

The Artery Wall: The Structure Beneath the Lining

Plaque develops within the wall. It may grow outward for years before causing a severe narrowing. A fixed narrowing can restrict blood flow; a change at a plaque's surface can trigger a sudden clot.

The Microcirculation: The Delivery System

Beyond the large coronary arteries lies a network of vessels too small to see on an ordinary angiogram. These vessels widen and narrow from moment to moment so oxygen delivery matches the heart's workload. They may fail to widen normally or may spasm even when the large arteries look open.

Flow in Action: Supply Must Meet Demand

Think of a two-lane road. At three in the morning, traffic moves easily; at five in the evening, it jams. The road has not changed. Demand has.

At rest, the heart may receive enough blood even when an artery is moderately narrowed. During exercise or stress, it needs more oxygen. The large arteries must deliver more blood, the lining must regulate that response, and the smallest vessels must widen downstream. If one part cannot respond, supply may fall short of demand, causing angina: chest discomfort or related symptoms when the heart muscle is not receiving enough oxygen-rich blood.

Beyond the Narrowing

Three questions before deciding what a narrowing means

THE PIPE PICTURE

Useful, but incomplete

How narrow does the artery look?

An anatomy question.

WIDEN THE VIEW →

THE FLOW MODEL

Adds function + context

What is present?
What is it doing?
What does it mean here?

THE THREE FLOW QUESTIONS

1 ANATOMY

What is present?

What do tests show about plaque and structure?

LIMIT: Anatomy alone cannot show whether a finding explains symptoms.

2 FUNCTION

What is it doing?

Does the narrowing limit blood flow? Can vessels respond?

LIMIT: Function alone cannot define future risk.

3 CONTEXT + GOAL

What does it mean here?

How urgent is the problem? What matters to this person?

LIMIT: No test predicts exactly what will happen.

Figure 3.2 · Beyond the Narrowing. The three Flow questions place anatomy, function, symptoms, overall risk, and treatment goals in the same decision.

The Same Narrowing, Different Decisions

The first, whom I will call Maria, has a 50 percent narrowing in one coronary artery. The anatomy tells us what is present; the next question is what the narrowing is doing.

A pressure measurement performed during angiography shows that the narrowing is not significantly limiting blood flow. Maria also has diabetes, a family history of early heart disease, and a high ApoB level, which reflects the number of potentially plaque-forming particles in her blood. Based on that flow measurement and in routine care, a stent for the narrowing would not be expected to help her feel better or prevent a future event; her overall risk calls for stronger prevention throughout the cardiovascular system.

David's angiogram shows the same 50 percent narrowing. In his case, the physiology test shows that it significantly limits blood flow and that the finding fits his persistent angina with activity despite appropriate medication. After discussing the options, we decide together to proceed with a stent to improve blood flow and relieve his symptoms.

The picture was the same. The meaning was not.

FLOW TRUTH

The choice is almost never stent or prevention. Everyone with plaque-related artery disease needs evidence-based prevention. Selected patients also need a procedure to restore blood flow. The Flow questions clarify what each treatment is being asked to accomplish.

Questions to Bring to Your Visit

At a visit, ask more than how narrow an artery looks. Ask what the test was designed to show and what decision the result changes.

- What did this test find, and what can it not rule out?
- Is a specific narrowing limiting blood flow or explaining my symptoms?
- What are the reasonable treatment options, and what is each meant to accomplish?
- What does my overall plaque burden or risk mean for prevention?
- Which new or changing symptoms require urgent care?

That is the sharper view: anatomy, blood flow, symptoms, and risk seen together. The next part turns to the forces that shape all four over a lifetime.

FLOW TAKEAWAY · CHAPTER 3

A narrowing percentage is a starting point. Ask what is present, what it is doing, and what it means here. Prevention protects the entire arterial system. When a procedure is proposed, ask whether its goal is to save heart muscle during an emergency, relieve persistent symptoms in selected stable disease, or improve outcomes in a selected high-risk anatomic or clinical situation.

PART II

What Shapes Your Flow

BIOLOGY

Life stage, inheritance, sleep, and access to care meet in the same arterial system.

CHAPTER 4

Five Major Drivers of Cardiovascular Risk

Early in my career, I placed a stent in a fellow physician, someone who had spent decades teaching other people how to protect their hearts. He knew every threat in this chapter cold. Every number, every guideline, every study. His arteries did not care.

That case stayed with me because it challenged a quiet bargain many of us make: knowing enough will keep us safe. Unfortunately, it will not. Arteries respond to what they experience year after year, not what a person knows.

A single narrowing is only one part of long-term risk. I begin with five common, changeable drivers: high blood pressure; LDL cholesterol and plaque-forming particles; diabetes or high blood sugar; tobacco exposure; and physical inactivity or excess abdominal fat. I then consider age, known disease, kidney health, inherited risk, pregnancy history or premature menopause, and access to care. The priorities differ from person to person. I want to know which risks matter most now and which changes are both safe and possible.

FLOW TRUTH

Long-term risk reflects exposures that accumulate and interact over time. Many can be lowered or treated; others reflect genetics, illness, and circumstances beyond a person's control.

Risk Factors Work Together

These risks can interact over time, but
none determines any one person's future.

MAJOR MODIFIABLE DRIVERS

LDL cholesterol and plaque-forming particles
More circulating particles mean more chances to enter the artery wall.

High blood pressure
Repeated pressure can strain the artery lining.

Diabetes or high blood sugar
Metabolic stress can damage vessels and speed plaque growth.

Tobacco exposure
Smoke and vaping aerosols can injure vessels and promote clotting.

Physical inactivity and excess abdominal fat
These can worsen blood pressure, the body's response to insulin, inflammation, and fitness.

↓

CAN INTERACT AND CONTRIBUTE TO

Artery lining stress	Inflammation and plaque growth	Flow problems or clot formation

RISK CAN ALSO BE AMPLIFIED BY

- Poor sleep or untreated sleep apnea
- Chronic kidney disease
- Long-term inflammatory disease
- Chronic stress

Figure 4.1 · Cardiovascular Risk Drivers and Amplifiers. Major modifiable risks can act together over time. Poor sleep, kidney disease, inflammatory disease, and chronic stress can intensify their effects.

These drivers can reinforce one another. High blood pressure, diabetes, tobacco exposure, and ApoB-containing particles can stress or injure the same arterial system over the same years. The first priority differs from one person to the next.

Nutrition shapes several of these drivers, including blood pressure, LDL and ApoB, blood sugar, and body composition. Patients often ask me what they should eat, and the honest answer is more useful than a rigid list. The overall pattern matters more than a perfect menu. The strongest guidance favors more vegetables, fruit, beans, whole grains, nuts, seeds, and other minimally processed foods; unsaturated fats in place of saturated fats; less sodium and added sugar; and fewer processed meats and ultraprocessed foods.

"Ultraprocessed" is an imperfect category, and a packaged food is not automatically a poor choice. Frozen vegetables, canned beans, plain yogurt, and whole-grain bread can all make a plan more practical. Culture, budget, access, allergies, kidney disease, diabetes, heart failure, and medicines change the details. The Toolkit's What Should I Eat? A Practical Flow Guide offers a starting plate you can adapt and repeat. Sleep, stress, kidney health, inherited risk, and access to care can influence the same drivers as well.

How Clinicians Turn Risk Factors Into a Plan

A risk factor is one part of the picture. A risk estimate combines several factors to approximate the chance of a cardiovascular event over a defined period. For adults ages 30 to 79 without known cardiovascular disease, the PREVENT equations estimate 10-year risk. In younger adults, a 30-year estimate can make the importance of long exposure easier to see.

The time horizon matters. A younger adult can have a low 10-year estimate while years of high LDL or blood pressure quietly build long-term risk. An older adult often has a higher near-term estimate partly because age itself carries risk. The calculation starts the conversation; the patient's history, priorities, and time horizon complete it.

Known plaque-related cardiovascular disease changes the starting point. A prior heart attack, an ischemic stroke from blocked blood flow to the brain, or peripheral artery disease causing symptoms from poor limb circulation already signals high risk. A prevention calculator is not needed to prove it.

EVIDENCE IN CONTEXT 4.1

What a Risk Reduction Actually Means

A practical way to read risk estimates and trial results

THE CORE IDEA

Risk estimates and trial results describe groups over a defined period. They do not forecast exactly what will happen to one person. Ask about absolute benefit as well as relative benefit.

STARTING RISK	AFTER A 25% RELATIVE REDUCTION	ABSOLUTE DIFFERENCE
20 in 100	15 in 100	5 fewer in 100
4 in 100	3 in 100	1 fewer in 100

WHAT THIS MEANS

The same proportional effect can produce very different absolute benefits because the starting risk is different.

IMPORTANT LIMIT

A risk estimate does not replace known disease or capture every risk-enhancing clue. A strong family history, elevated lipoprotein(a), or Lp(a), pregnancy complications or premature menopause, chronic inflammatory disease, and selected imaging findings may change the plan. A low 10-year estimate in a younger adult may also hide the importance of decades of exposure.

The Five Drivers

1. High Blood Pressure

High blood pressure often causes no symptoms, which is why repeated measurements matter. One reading is a snapshot. Repeated office measurements or a correctly collected home series show the pattern more reliably. Sustained high pressure stresses artery walls and raises the risk of heart attack, stroke, kidney disease, and heart failure, meaning the heart cannot pump or fill normally. Treating it lowers cardiovascular risk.

2. LDL and ApoB-Containing Particles

Most patients first see LDL-C on a standard lipid panel. LDL-C estimates how much cholesterol is carried inside LDL particles. ApoB is the particle count in practical terms: because each potentially plaque-forming particle carries one ApoB protein, the blood level estimates how many are circulating. The two numbers often move together, but they can diverge, especially with diabetes or high triglycerides.

Risk reflects both particle number and years of exposure. Lifestyle supports the whole prevention plan; medication is often needed when overall risk is higher. Lowering LDL lowers cardiovascular events.

EVIDENCE SNAPSHOT 4.2

Lower LDL, Fewer Cardiovascular Events

FOURIER · NEW ENGLAND JOURNAL OF MEDICINE, 2017

WHAT WAS STUDIED

FOURIER randomly assigned 27,564 adults with established plaque-related cardiovascular disease who were already taking a statin cholesterol-lowering medicine to evolocumab, an injectable LDL-lowering medicine, or placebo. Median follow-up was 2.2 years.

WHAT RESEARCHERS FOUND

Median LDL-C fell from 92 mg/dL at baseline to 30 mg/dL with evolocumab at 48 weeks. The primary combined outcome fell from 11.3% to 9.8%; cardiovascular death, heart attack, or stroke fell from 7.4% to 5.9%. Each absolute difference was 1.5 fewer events per 100 people.

WHAT THIS MEANS

Lowering LDL further reduced cardiovascular events in people who already had established disease and were receiving statin therapy.

IMPORTANT LIMIT

Relative risk fell 15% for the primary outcome and 20% for the key secondary outcome. Each absolute difference was 1.5 percentage points over a median of 2.2 years. Cardiovascular death alone was not significantly lower.

3. Diabetes and Metabolic Health

Diabetes develops when blood sugar remains too high because the body makes too little insulin, responds poorly to it, or both. Insulin resistance is that reduced response to insulin. Over time, both raise cardiovascular risk and affect large and small vessels. A hemoglobin A1c blood test estimates average blood sugar over about three months. Prediabetes is a reason to review blood pressure, triglycerides, activity, sleep, weight when relevant, and the overall prevention plan together.

4. Smoking and Vaping

Cigarette smoking is a major, well-established cause of cardiovascular disease. Vaping is not harmless: its aerosol can contain nicotine, ultrafine particles, metals, and other chemicals, and human studies show adverse short-term effects on blood pressure and blood-vessel function. Because these products are newer, their long-term cardiovascular event risk is still being defined.

Stopping either exposure matters. For cigarette smoking, proven ways to help people quit include nicotine replacement, varenicline, bupropion, counseling, and quitlines. A clinician can also help build a plan for stopping vaping. Many people need more than one attempt, and that is not failure.

5. Physical Inactivity, Low Fitness, and Visceral Fat

Regular physical activity improves fitness, blood pressure, insulin sensitivity, and overall cardiovascular health. Long periods of inactivity work in the opposite direction. Activity and body composition are different, but both can shape metabolic health.

Fat stored around the internal organs, called visceral fat, is associated with insulin resistance, higher triglycerides, fatty liver disease, and inflammation. Body size or appearance alone does not define a person's risk. Assessment should focus on health measures, function, and a plan that is realistic and free of blame.

Other Findings That Change the Plan

Certain findings change the plan because they signal higher cardiovascular risk.

Table 4.1 · Findings That Can Change the Plan

Clinical clue	Why it changes the conversation
Known atherosclerotic cardiovascular disease (ASCVD)	A prior heart attack, ischemic stroke, peripheral artery disease, or established coronary disease shifts care from estimating risk to treating known disease.
Chronic kidney disease	Reduced kidney function or albumin (a protein) in the urine raises risk and can change medicine choice and monitoring.
Inherited risk	Early disease in close relatives, inherited very high LDL, or elevated lipoprotein(a), also called Lp(a), may justify earlier prevention.
Life-stage, inflammatory, and cancer history	Pregnancy complications, premature menopause, chronic inflammation, chest radiation, or cancer treatment that affects the cardiovascular system can change follow-up.

Risk Is Individual, and Access to Care Matters

A risk calculator cannot see whether a patient can afford a medicine, reach the clinic, or find healthy food and a safe place to exercise. Those barriers belong in the medical conversation.

Stress, Sleep, and Untreated Sleep Apnea

Chronic stress and disrupted sleep can worsen blood pressure, glucose control, appetite, inflammation, and recovery. Obstructive sleep apnea repeatedly narrows or closes the upper airway during sleep and interrupts breathing. Untreated, it can contribute to difficult-to-control blood pressure and is associated with atrial fibrillation (AFib), an irregular heart rhythm, stroke, heart failure, and coronary disease. These factors can intensify the five drivers or make them harder to control. Chapter 7 explains testing and treatment.

Putting the Drivers Together

Ask which measurements matter for you and what decision each will change. For many adults, the starting picture includes a properly measured blood-pressure pattern, a standard lipid panel, and a blood-sugar assessment. ApoB can clarify particle number in selected patients. Lipoprotein(a), or Lp(a), is a mostly inherited cholesterol-related particle and should be measured at least once in adulthood. Kidney function and urine protein matter for many people as well. A test is most useful when its result has a decision attached to it.

I start with anything immediately dangerous, then move to the largest untreated risks. Choose changes that are safe and realistic. For each recommendation, know what it is meant to improve, how you and your care team will judge whether it is working, and when you will revisit it. Practical barriers can change the plan.

FLOW PRACTICE · START A BLOOD-PRESSURE PATTERN

If home blood-pressure monitoring is part of your plan, take one correctly collected reading and record it. Do not judge control from one number; begin the pattern.

FLOW TAKEAWAY · CHAPTER 4

Cardiovascular risk is cumulative, interactive, and personal. Focus first on the largest risks that are both important and changeable. Improving several major drivers usually matters more than perfecting one number while ignoring the rest.

Use next: Flow Tool 10, My Cardiovascular Risk Snapshot.

CHAPTER 5

Women's Flow: Patterns Too Often Missed

One woman I still think about had visited three emergency departments in a year for exertional chest pressure. Each time, an electrocardiogram (ECG) showed no electrical pattern suggesting reduced blood flow to the heart muscle or injury, and troponin testing showed no heart-muscle injury. Stress testing did not show a large area of reduced blood flow. Each result was reassuring, but none explained why symptoms kept returning. When her large coronary arteries were finally pictured, they showed no major blockage.

By the time she reached my office, she had stopped trusting herself. She apologized for taking up my time.

But her pattern was real: pressure with effort, relief with rest, and symptoms that were worse in cold weather. Further testing showed that blood flow through her coronary circulation could not rise normally when her heart worked harder. The problem was not a major blockage in one of the large surface arteries. It was dysfunction in the heart's smallest vessels, which were not widening enough to meet demand. This is called coronary microvascular dysfunction.

She was relieved to have an explanation and understandably angry that it had taken a year to find one.

Heart disease remains the leading cause of death for women in the United States. Women develop the same plaque, major coronary blockages, and heart attacks described in the earlier chapters.

But women are more likely than men to have symptoms or evidence of reduced blood flow without a major blockage in the large coronary arteries. The explanation may lie in the small vessels, a temporary tightening called coronary spasm, plaque spread along a longer section of artery, or another condition entirely. Pregnancy, menopause, inflammatory disease, and certain cancer treatments can also add clues that a routine risk calculation may miss.

Chapter 4 described the major risk drivers that apply to everyone. This chapter adds the parts of a woman's history that can change when to look, what to measure, and what question to ask next.

FLOW TRUTH

Women can have the same large-artery disease as men. They can also have important symptoms when no major blockage is present. An angiogram without a major blockage narrows the question; it does not end the evaluation.

Why Women Are So Often Missed

Chest pressure or discomfort is the most common heart-attack symptom in women, just as it is in men. Women commonly report breathlessness, nausea, unusual fatigue, back or jaw discomfort, or sleep disturbance as well.

FLOW SAFETY · WHEN SYMPTOMS MAY BE AN EMERGENCY

New, worsening, or severe symptoms still require prompt evaluation. Use the Start Here emergency guidance rather than a prior reassuring test to decide that a new symptom is safe.

Sudden or severe chest pressure, especially with shortness of breath, sweating, nausea, or faintness, requires urgent evaluation. Call 911 for severe, rapidly worsening, or persistent symptoms that may represent an emergency.

Gaps in Care

Many cardiovascular tests answer a specific question. An ECG and serial troponin measurements look for acute electrical changes and heart-muscle injury. A stress test looks for a blood-flow problem under the conditions tested. An angiogram maps the large coronary arteries. None of those tests alone evaluates every possible cause of chest symptoms.

Anxiety, reflux, lung disease, anemia (reduced oxygen-carrying capacity in the blood), muscle or joint pain, and menopause can all cause or contribute to symptoms. Considering those possibilities is appropriate. The error is settling on one before the full pattern has been assessed.

Research has documented differences in how cardiovascular symptoms are recognized, investigated, and treated. Those gaps are not experienced equally. Race, income, geography, disability, language, and access to care can influence who is heard, who is tested, and who reaches specialty care.

Describe what brings the symptom on, what relieves it, how long it lasts, and whether the pattern is changing. Clinicians should make room for those questions. The burden of communication should not rest on the patient alone.

When the Large Arteries Do Not Explain the Symptoms

A coronary angiogram is a map of the large arteries on the heart's surface. It is excellent at finding a major narrowing or blockage. It does not directly show how the heart's microscopic vessels respond when demand rises.

Several mechanisms remain possible after no major blockage is found.

Coronary microvascular dysfunction can occur when the heart's smallest vessels do not widen enough as demand rises. Symptoms often appear with activity or emotional stress and improve with rest.

Coronary spasm is a different mechanism: a temporary abnormal tightening of a large surface artery or smaller vessels. It can occur at rest, including at night or early in the morning.

Diffuse or nonobstructive plaque means that plaque is present but does not form one tight blockage. It still matters for prevention. Whether it explains the symptoms requires clinical judgment and, sometimes, additional testing.

These mechanisms can overlap. A person may also have a cause outside the heart. Finding no major blockage narrows the field; it does not end the evaluation. Chapter 11 returns to this woman and explains how selected tests can help distinguish these mechanisms.

When Small Vessels Do Not Increase Blood Flow

The large coronary arteries may have no major blockage while the smallest vessels still fail to deliver enough blood when the heart works harder.

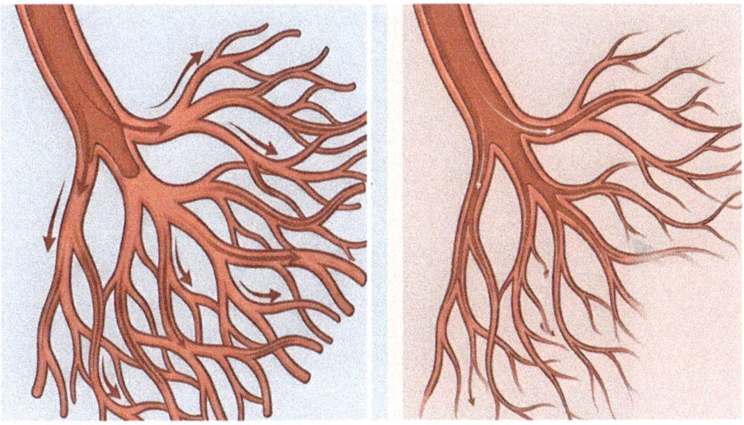

Normal response

Small vessels widen. Blood flow rises as the heart works harder.

Microvascular dysfunction

Small vessels do not widen enough - or may tighten. Blood flow may not rise enough.

> **No major blockage does not mean no coronary problem.**
>
> An angiogram maps the large arteries; it does not test how the smallest vessels work. Other tests can measure small-vessel function.

Figure 5.1 · When Small Vessels Do Not Increase Blood Flow. Coronary microvascular dysfunction can limit the normal rise in blood flow even when no major blockage is present in the large coronary arteries.

Risk Across the Life Course

Cardiovascular risk changes across a woman's life, and important clues are easy to miss on a standard intake form. Reproductive history, pregnancy complications, the timing and cause of menopause, polycystic ovary syndrome (PCOS), a hormonal and metabolic condition often linked with irregular periods and insulin resistance, autoimmune disease, and previous cancer treatment can all change how prevention is reviewed.

These clues are not predictions. They help identify when to take a closer look.

REPRODUCTIVE AND INFLAMMATORY HISTORY

Earlier clues matter

PCOS can involve irregular periods and insulin resistance. PCOS, lupus, and rheumatoid arthritis are cardiovascular clues.

PREGNANCY AND AFTER DELIVERY

Keep the history

High blood pressure or diabetes during pregnancy, delivery before 37 weeks, or heart-muscle weakness around childbirth should remain in your history.

MENOPAUSE

Recheck the risk factors

LDL-C, ApoB, blood pressure, sleep, body composition, and blood sugar can change. Menopause before age 40 is linked with higher long-term risk.

CANCER TREATMENT OR TREATMENT-RELATED MENOPAUSE

Treatment can change follow-up

Chest radiation, some cancer medicines, or treatment-related menopause can change the monitoring and prevention you need.

These clues can change when and how prevention is reviewed.

They do not determine any one woman's future.

Figure 5.2 · Cardiovascular Clues Across a Woman's Life. Reproductive, pregnancy, menopause, inflammatory, and treatment history can change when prevention is reviewed.

Pregnancy History and Future Cardiovascular Risk

Pregnancy places substantial additional demand on the heart and circulation. Certain pregnancy complications are associated with a higher risk of developing high blood pressure, diabetes, heart disease, heart failure, or stroke later in life.

The terminology can sound more complicated than it is:

- **Preeclampsia** is new high blood pressure after 20 weeks of pregnancy or soon after delivery, together with signs that organs such as the kidneys, liver, brain, or blood-clotting system are under stress.
- **Gestational hypertension** is new high blood pressure that begins during pregnancy without the other findings required for a diagnosis of preeclampsia.
- **Gestational diabetes** is high blood sugar first diagnosed during pregnancy.
- **Preterm delivery** means delivery before 37 completed weeks of pregnancy.

None of these complications guarantees future heart disease. They identify a history that should remain visible after the pregnancy is over. A complication may reveal an underlying susceptibility, contribute to later risk, or do both.

Keep pregnancy complications in the permanent medical history, even when the pregnancy was decades ago and the problem appeared to resolve.

After gestational diabetes, a 75-gram oral glucose tolerance test is recommended 4 to 12 weeks after delivery, followed by lifelong blood-sugar screening every 1 to 3 years. After preeclampsia or gestational hypertension, follow the postpartum blood-pressure plan and confirm who will monitor long-term cardiovascular risk.

> **FLOW TRUTH**
> A pregnancy complication is not destiny, but it should not disappear from the medical record when the pregnancy ends.

Before Pregnancy, or If Pregnancy Is Possible

Some cardiovascular medicines require a different plan during pregnancy. Abruptly stopping treatment can also be dangerous.

If you are planning a pregnancy or could become pregnant, review your heart or vascular condition and every prescription, over-the-counter medicine, and supplement with your clinicians before conception when possible. Tell prescribers promptly about pregnancy, pregnancy plans, or breastfeeding. Do not stop a cardiovascular medicine on your own.

Women with significant heart or vascular disease may benefit from coordinated care by cardiology and high-risk pregnancy specialists. This is often called a cardio-obstetrics team or Pregnancy Heart Team.

Menopause Is a Time to Review Risk

Perimenopause is the transition leading up to menopause, when menstrual cycles and hormone levels begin to change. Aging and the menopause transition occur together, so their effects cannot always be separated cleanly. Going through menopause does not by itself cause cardiovascular disease, but cardiovascular risk often rises during this stage.

LDL-C and the ApoB particle count can rise. Blood pressure, blood sugar, body composition, sleep, and activity often change as well. This makes the menopause transition a useful time to review the prevention plan rather than waiting for a problem to appear.

Natural menopause before age 40 is called premature menopause and is associated with higher long-term cardiovascular risk. Menopause caused at a young age by removal of the ovaries, radiation, chemotherapy, or other treatment may also justify an earlier review of blood pressure, cholesterol, blood sugar, tobacco exposure, sleep, activity, and family history.

New chest pressure, shortness of breath, palpitations, or declining exercise tolerance should not automatically be attributed to menopause. Menopause provides context; it is not a diagnosis.

Systemic menopausal hormone therapy can be appropriate for selected symptoms after an individualized discussion. It should not be started solely to prevent heart disease.

The balance of benefits and risks depends on age, timing, the medicine and dose, how it is taken, and a woman's history of blood clots, stroke, heart or blood-vessel disease, and cancer. Hormone therapy does not replace indicated treatment of high blood pressure, cholesterol, diabetes, or tobacco exposure.

Other History That Can Change the Assessment

Polycystic ovary syndrome, usually shortened to PCOS, is a hormonal and metabolic condition that can cause irregular periods and is often associated with insulin resistance. For cardiovascular care, PCOS is a reason to review blood pressure, blood sugar, cholesterol, weight, sleep, and other risk factors together.

Lupus and rheumatoid arthritis are autoimmune diseases, meaning the immune system mistakenly attacks the body's own tissues. Their long-term inflammation can accelerate vascular disease. Prior chest radiation and certain cancer medicines can also affect the heart, valves, heart muscle, or arteries years later. Tell your clinician what treatment you received and when, even if it now feels like distant history.

Conditions That Require a Different Path

Not every heart attack in women begins with ordinary plaque rupture and a clot. Finding the cause matters because testing and treatment may differ.

Spontaneous coronary artery dissection, or SCAD, is bleeding or separation within the wall of a coronary artery. The affected artery wall can squeeze the normal blood channel and cause a heart attack. SCAD is not the same process as ordinary plaque rupture.

MINOCA stands for myocardial infarction with nonobstructive coronary arteries. In plain language, testing confirms a heart attack, but an angiogram does not show a major blockage that fully explains it. MINOCA is a working diagnosis, not the end of the evaluation. The next step is to identify the underlying cause.

Peripartum cardiomyopathy is new weakness of the heart's main pumping chamber that develops near the end of pregnancy or in the months after delivery when no other cause explains it. Fatigue, swelling, and shortness of breath can occur in normal pregnancy, which is one reason this condition is sometimes missed.

New or progressive shortness of breath, difficulty breathing while lying flat, rapidly worsening swelling, chest pain, fainting, or a sustained fast heartbeat during or after pregnancy deserve prompt medical evaluation. Call 911 for severe breathlessness, chest pain, fainting, or rapidly worsening symptoms.

Takotsubo syndrome is a sudden, usually temporary weakening of the heart muscle that can resemble a heart attack. It is discussed further in Chapter 15.

FLOW TAKEAWAY · CHAPTER 5

Women can develop plaque, major blockages, and heart attacks, just as men can. They can also have small-vessel dysfunction, coronary spasm, or acute heart injury from a different mechanism. Pregnancy, menopause, inflammatory disease, and treatment history can change when prevention should begin. When symptoms persist after reassuring testing, ask what the test made less likely, what it did not assess, and what question remains unanswered.

Use next: Flow Tool 5, Women's and Pregnancy-Related Cardiovascular History Guide.

CHAPTER 6

Inherited Risk: Family History, Genes, and Lp(a)

If heart disease seems to run through your family, you may have asked a question I hear every week: "Is this going to happen to me?"

No family history, blood test, or genetic result can tell you exactly whether you will have a heart attack. Inherited information changes probability, not certainty. Its value is practical: it can change when you look, what you measure, how strongly you treat changeable risks, and which relatives may benefit from testing.

When a parent or sibling has had an early heart attack, I begin prevention sooner and look more carefully for inherited conditions. These may include familial hypercholesterolemia, an inherited cause of very high LDL, or elevated lipoprotein(a), written Lp(a), a mostly inherited cholesterol-related particle. I also pay attention to a confirmed disease-causing result on a clinical genetic test. The point is not to prove that an event is inevitable. It is to avoid missing a risk that can be measured or treated.

Inherited risk changes the starting point. It can change when common risk drivers should be measured, how seriously an abnormal result should be taken, and which relatives may need testing.

> **FLOW TRUTH**
>
> Inherited risk is not a countdown clock. Its value lies in changing the plan: when to look, what to measure, how to manage treatable risks, and whom else to test.

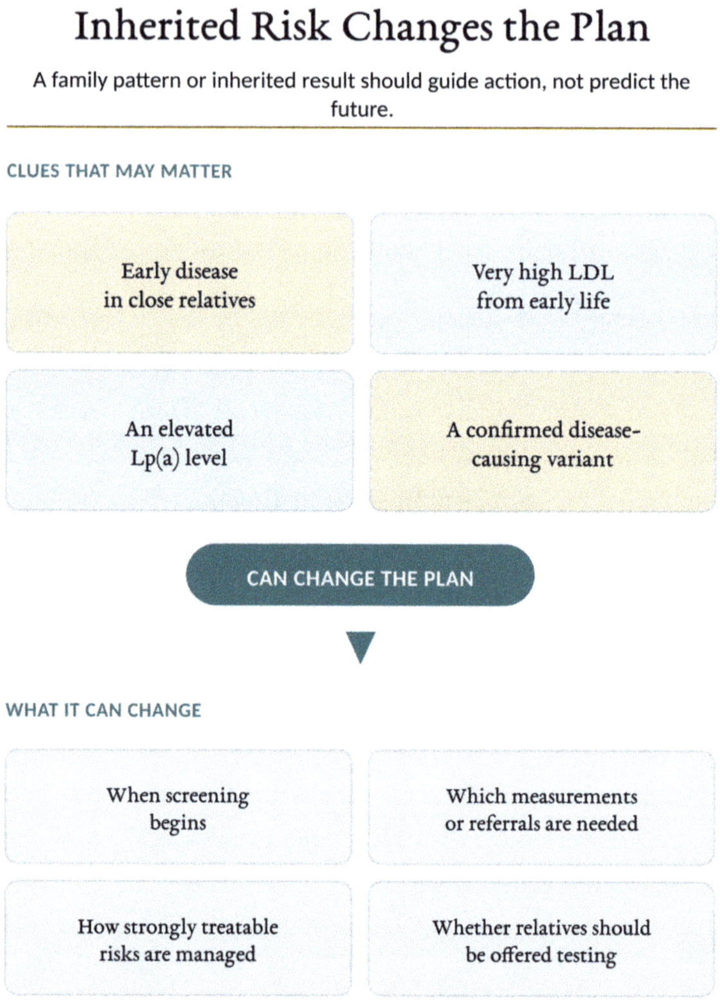

Figure 6.1 · Inherited Risk Changes the Plan. Family history and inherited findings can change when to screen, what to measure, and whom else to test.

Family History: A Signal, Not a Verdict

Family history is sometimes treated as though it were a genetic test. In practice, it is a useful clue, even when the details are incomplete or uncertain.

Parents, siblings, and children are called first-degree relatives. You do not need to know the exact medical diagnosis. Start with what happened, which relative was affected, and approximately how old the person was. The following patterns are especially important to report:

- A heart attack, an ischemic stroke (a stroke caused by blocked blood flow to the brain), or symptomatic peripheral artery disease (poor circulation in an arm or leg) before age 55 in a father, brother, or son, or before age 65 in a mother, sister, or daughter.
- Several close relatives with cardiovascular disease at unusually young ages.
- Very high LDL-C, known familial hypercholesterolemia (an inherited cause of very high LDL), or markedly elevated Lp(a), a mostly inherited cholesterol-related particle, in the family.
- Unexplained sudden death, heart-muscle disease, or a serious inherited rhythm disorder in a close relative.
- An aortic aneurysm or dissection (an abnormal enlargement or tear involving the aorta, the body's main artery), especially at a young age.
- A confirmed disease-causing result on a clinical genetic test for a heart or aortic condition in a close relative.

Those age cutoffs are clinical conventions for "premature" disease, not a border between meaningful and meaningless history. An event shortly after a cutoff may still matter, especially when several relatives are affected.

When available, death certificates, procedure reports, cholesterol results, and genetic reports can clarify the pattern.

A relative's smoking, diabetes, or other risk factors do not make the family history irrelevant. Inherited and acquired risks can operate at the same time.

Familial Hypercholesterolemia: High LDL From Early Life

One inherited condition deserves particular attention because it is common, underdiagnosed, and treatable.

Familial hypercholesterolemia, or FH, causes very high LDL exposure from early life. It is not simply a high cholesterol result today. It reflects years of LDL particles entering the artery wall, often beginning in childhood.

In an adult, an untreated LDL-C of 190 mg/dL or higher is considered severe hypercholesterolemia and should trigger a closer evaluation. The number raises suspicion; by itself, it does not prove FH.

Clinicians look for a pattern:

- LDL-C that was already high earlier in life
- Early cardiovascular disease in the patient or family
- Very high LDL-C in close relatives
- Cholesterol deposits in tendons, called tendon xanthomas

They also check whether another health condition or medicine could explain the LDL elevation.

Bring older untreated cholesterol results if you have them. A current value obtained while taking medication may hide the degree of earlier exposure.

A genetic change classified as pathogenic or likely pathogenic is known or strongly suspected to cause disease. Finding one in an FH-related gene can confirm an inherited cause and make family screening more precise. A negative test does not rule FH out; some people meet clinical criteria even when no causative variant is found.

Once FH is recognized, treatment should begin early and remain consistent. Parents, siblings, and children may benefit from cascade screening, which means testing relatives step by step after one person is diagnosed. Children should receive age-appropriate evaluation through their clinician rather than waiting until adulthood.

Lp(a): An Inherited Risk You Can Measure

Lipoprotein(a), written Lp(a) and pronounced "L-P-little-a," is a cholesterol-carrying particle whose level is determined largely by inheritance. Most people with an elevated level have no symptoms, and the result is not included in a standard cholesterol panel.

High Lp(a) is associated with plaque-related cardiovascular disease and calcific aortic stenosis, a narrowing of the heart's main outflow valve. A person can have high Lp(a) even when LDL-C looks acceptable.

The 2026 U.S. dyslipidemia guideline recommends measuring Lp(a) at least once in adulthood. An Lp(a) level is relatively stable, so repeated testing is often unnecessary unless a specific clinical reason exists. Risk rises continuously with the level rather than changing suddenly at a single cutoff.

Why the Units Matter

Laboratories report Lp(a) in either nmol/L or mg/dL. Nanomoles per liter estimates particle concentration; milligrams per deciliter reports mass.

Because Lp(a) particles differ in size, the units are not directly interchangeable. The paired guideline thresholds are approximate reference points, not a conversion formula, and there is no reliable universal way to convert between them.

What an Elevated Result Changes

An elevated Lp(a) does not prove that a blockage is present, predict when an event will occur, or automatically dictate one medication. It changes the overall risk discussion.

The practical response is usually to manage the risks that can be changed more intensively: LDL-C and the ApoB particle count, blood pressure, diabetes, tobacco exposure, activity, and the rest of the prevention plan. Statins do not meaningfully lower Lp(a), but they can still lower overall cardiovascular risk by reducing LDL-related exposure.

Lifestyle changes usually have little effect on the Lp(a) number itself. Their benefit comes from improving the rest of the risk profile: LDL-C or ApoB, blood pressure, blood sugar, activity, tobacco exposure, sleep, and weight when relevant.

As this book went to press, no medication was approved by the U.S. Food and Drug Administration (FDA) specifically to lower Lp(a) and reduce events. Several targeted therapies were in clinical trials. For now, a high Lp(a) level can sharpen the overall prevention plan, support more intensive management of changeable risks, and, when the level is high, identify relatives who should be offered testing.

Lp(a) is usually stable, so routine repeat testing is generally unnecessary unless a clinician has a specific reason to repeat it.

Genetic Testing: When It Clarifies the Plan

A clinical genetic test should answer a defined question. It may be useful when the history suggests FH, an inherited heart-muscle disorder, a serious rhythm condition, an inherited aortic disorder, or another specific syndrome.

Testing without a clear question is more likely to produce uncertainty that does not improve care. Genetic counseling can help select the right test, explain what it can and cannot find, and plan how a meaningful result should be shared with relatives.

How to Read the Result

Genetic reports generally use three important categories:

- **Pathogenic or likely pathogenic:** Evidence supports the conclusion that the variant causes or contributes to disease. The result still may not predict exactly when disease will appear or how severe it will be.
- **Variant of uncertain significance, or VUS:** The evidence is not settled. A VUS should not, by itself, diagnose a condition, change treatment, or be used to test relatives as though it were definitive.
- **Negative:** No disease-causing variant was found in the genes examined. This is not always an "all clear." Current testing does not identify every inherited cause, and some conditions can be diagnosed clinically.

Variant classifications can change as evidence grows. Keep a copy of the complete report and ask who is responsible for notifying you if its interpretation changes.

Consumer DNA Tests

Consumer DNA reports and clinical genetic tests are not interchangeable. Some consumer tests examine only selected variants, and third-party interpretations of downloaded raw data can be wrong.

Any result that could change medical care should be confirmed in an appropriate clinical laboratory and interpreted alongside the person's medical and family history.

Polygenic Risk Scores

Most coronary disease is not caused by one powerful variant. Thousands of common variants can each nudge risk by a small amount. A polygenic risk score combines selected variants to estimate how a person's inherited susceptibility compares with that of others.

The 2026 dyslipidemia guideline lists high polygenic risk, if measured, as a risk-enhancing factor. A score may sometimes help when a prevention decision remains uncertain, but routine testing is not established for everyone.

Polygenic scores do not diagnose disease or predict an event. Their performance can differ across ancestry groups. A low score should never overrule known disease, severe LDL elevation, elevated Lp(a), or a compelling family history.

EVIDENCE SNAPSHOT 6.1

At High Genetic Risk, Lifestyle Still Mattered

KHERA ET AL. · NEW ENGLAND JOURNAL OF MEDICINE, 2016

WHAT WAS STUDIED

Researchers examined genetic risk and four lifestyle factors in 55,685 participants across three prospective cohorts and one cross-sectional study. A favorable lifestyle meant meeting at least three of four criteria: no current smoking, no obesity, regular physical activity, and a healthier diet.

WHAT RESEARCHERS FOUND

Among participants in the highest genetic-risk group, a favorable lifestyle was associated with 46% lower relative coronary risk than an unfavorable lifestyle (hazard ratio, 0.54; 95% CI, 0.47–0.63). In one cohort, standardized 10-year event rates were 5.1% versus 10.7%.

WHAT THIS MEANS

Even in the highest genetic-risk group, lifestyle remained associated with a substantial difference in coronary risk.

> **IMPORTANT LIMIT**
> This was observational, so it cannot prove that the lifestyle profile caused the entire difference or erased inherited risk. The score used variants available in 2016 and is not equivalent to every current or consumer genetic test.

Turn Inherited Risk Into a Family Plan

Inherited information becomes useful when it changes a decision. Ask:

- Does my family history change when screening should begin?
- Have I had Lp(a) measured at least once?
- Does my highest untreated LDL-C raise concern for FH?
- Would clinical genetic testing or genetic counseling clarify anything?
- Which relatives should be tested, with what test, and at what age?

Create a simple family map that records the relative, the diagnosis, and the age when it occurred. Update it when new information appears. If a meaningful result is found, share the actual report rather than relying on memory or a verbal summary.

The goal is not to predict a family's future. It is to make earlier prevention possible.

FLOW PRACTICE · MAP THE FAMILY HISTORY

Write down which close relatives had heart or vascular disease and approximately how old they were. Bring either the list or the Family Flow Map to your next prevention visit.

FLOW TAKEAWAY · CHAPTER 6

Inherited risk is not a forecast. It tells you when to look sooner, what to measure, how intensively to manage changeable risks, and which relatives may benefit from testing. A high-risk result does not erase the value of prevention, and a reassuring result does not erase known disease or a strong clinical history.

Use next: Flow Tool 7, Family Flow Map.

CHAPTER 7

Sleep, Obstructive Sleep Apnea, and the Heart

If your blood pressure stays high despite treatment or atrial fibrillation keeps returning, I ask a question that can be surprising: How are you sleeping? Sometimes a partner describes the pattern first: loud snoring, then a long silence, then a gasp.

We often assess heart health in daylight: a blood-pressure reading in the office, a morning cholesterol panel, a treadmill test. But for many people, an important cardiovascular stress happens at night and goes unnoticed for years.

Sleep problems take several forms. Too little sleep, irregular sleep, insomnia, and obstructive sleep apnea (OSA) can overlap. OSA deserves separate attention because it is a breathing disorder with its own tests and treatments.

Sleep Health Is More Than Apnea

Sleep duration, regularity, and continuity all matter. Most adults do best when they have a regular opportunity for seven to nine hours, although individual need varies and work, caregiving, pain, housing, stress, or illness often make that difficult. The goal is not perfect sleep or another score to feel guilty about.

Insomnia and OSA can occur together, but they are different disorders. Insomnia is persistent difficulty falling asleep, staying asleep, or returning to sleep despite adequate opportunity; OSA is repeated upper-airway obstruction. They require separate evaluation and sometimes separate treatment. When fatigue persists, blood pressure stays high, or mood or recovery does not improve, I ask about both.

What Happens While You Sleep

Obstructive sleep apnea occurs when the upper airway repeatedly narrows or closes during sleep while the body is still trying to breathe. With each obstruction, the chest pulls against a closed airway, oxygen may fall, and the nervous system releases a burst of stress signals that can raise heart rate and blood pressure. Breathing resumes, often with a gasp or snort, and the cycle starts again. Most people do not remember these brief awakenings; they know only that they wake unrefreshed.

How Obstructive Sleep Apnea Stresses the Heart

Each breathing pause can trigger this cycle—many times a night.

1 Airway narrows or closes

Airflow slows or stops.

2 Oxygen may fall; the brain briefly wakes

Airflow restarts—often without you knowing.

3 Stress response surges

Heart rate and blood pressure rise.

4 Sleep becomes fragmented

Repeated arousals reduce restorative sleep.

WHY THIS MATTERS

Untreated sleep apnea is associated with high blood pressure, atrial fibrillation, stroke, and heart failure. These associations do not predict what will happen to one person.

TESTING AND TREATMENT ARE INDIVIDUALIZED

Testing

A sleep study shows whether apnea is present and how severe it is.

Treatment

Options may include airway-pressure therapy, a custom oral appliance, weight management, position changes, or surgery.

Figure 7.1 · How Obstructive Sleep Apnea Stresses the Heart. Obstructive sleep apnea can repeatedly lower oxygen, fragment sleep, and raise heart rate and blood pressure.

Your significant other may notice loud snoring, pauses, choking, or sudden silence. The person with OSA may notice morning headaches, dry mouth, poor concentration, irritability, insomnia, or daytime fatigue. Not everyone is sleepy, and not everyone fits the familiar image of an older man who snores and carries excess weight.

Why the Heart Cares

OSA is associated with high blood pressure, especially pressure that remains high despite several medicines, and with atrial fibrillation, heart failure, stroke, and coronary disease. Repeated oxygen changes and stress-response surges may help explain why blood pressure or a rhythm problem remains difficult to control. That is why sleep belongs in a heart-care plan.

How Sleep Apnea Is Diagnosed

A home sleep apnea test can diagnose OSA in many adults whose symptoms suggest moderate-to-severe disease and whose overall health makes home testing appropriate. It measures breathing, oxygen, and other signals while you sleep in your own bed. It is convenient, and usually the first test to order when screening for OSA

A laboratory study preferred if the home sleep study was equivocal, or the picture includes significant heart or lung disease, nerve or muscle weakness, prior stroke, chronic opioid use, severe insomnia, suspected underbreathing during sleep, or suspected central sleep apnea, in which breathing effort briefly stops.

Ask your clinician whether OSA could be part of the picture if you have loud habitual snoring, witnessed breathing pauses, choking or gasping, unexplained fatigue, daytime sleepiness, or morning headaches. Also raise the question if you have atrial fibrillation, difficult-to-control blood pressure, obesity or a larger neck size, prior stroke, or heart failure. OSA can occur in people who are not overweight, and women may report insomnia, fatigue, headache, or mood changes rather than dramatic snoring.

How to Read a Sleep-Study Report

A sleep-study report is more than a single number. Read the event count with the oxygen pattern, event type, symptoms, and study type.

Table 7.1 · How to Read a Sleep-Study Report

MEASURE	WHAT IT MEANS AND WHAT TO REMEMBER
AHI	The apnea-hypopnea index counts complete pauses and partial reductions per hour of actual sleep in a laboratory study. Mild is 5–14.9; moderate, 15–29.9; severe, 30 or more. Remember: The category does not capture every symptom or cardiovascular effect.
REI	The respiratory event index counts events per hour of recording time, commonly on a home test. Remember: Recording time may exceed actual sleep time, so REI can underestimate severity.
Oxygen pattern	Includes how low oxygen fell and how often drops occurred. Remember: The same AHI can accompany different oxygen exposure; a low reading may also reflect a poor signal.
Event pattern	Events may be obstructive or central and may cluster on the back or during dream sleep. Remember: The pattern may change treatment or prompt further evaluation.

A watch, ring, or consumer oxygen monitor may identify oxygen changes, snoring, or restless sleep, but it cannot confirm or exclude OSA. A clinician-ordered home test uses medically validated signals and is interpreted in context. If that study is negative or inconclusive and concern remains high, ask whether a laboratory study is appropriate.

What Treatment Can Realistically Do

Continuous positive airway pressure, or CPAP, keeps the airway open with gentle air pressure through a mask. Used consistently, it reliably reduces breathing interruptions, often reduces daytime sleepiness, and improves quality of life. It also lowers blood pressure modestly on average, although some people, particularly those with resistant hypertension, may see a larger benefit.

I explain CPAP by starting with what it reliably changes: airway obstruction, broken sleep, and often the sleepiness or mental fog that can linger the next day. The SAVE trial helps put those benefits in context.

EVIDENCE SNAPSHOT 7.1

What CPAP Has—and Has Not—Been Shown to Do

SAVE · NEW ENGLAND JOURNAL OF MEDICINE, 2016

WHAT WAS STUDIED

SAVE randomly assigned 2,717 adults aged 45 to 75 with moderate-to-severe obstructive sleep apnea and established coronary or cerebrovascular disease to CPAP plus usual care or usual care alone. Most participants had little daytime sleepiness.

WHAT RESEARCHERS FOUND

Over a mean of 3.7 years, the main cardiovascular outcome occurred in 17.0% of the CPAP group and 15.4% of the usual-care group (hazard ratio, 1.10; 95% CI, 0.91–1.32). CPAP reduced snoring and sleepiness and improved quality of life and mood.

WHAT THIS MEANS

Use CPAP to treat airway obstruction and improve sleepiness and quality of life while the rest of the cardiovascular plan continues.

> **IMPORTANT LIMIT**
> Average CPAP use was 3.3 hours per night, and most participants had minimal sleepiness. The trial therefore cannot fully answer what more consistent use or treatment in different OSA populations might do.

A treatment that sits unused beside the bed cannot help. If CPAP feels uncomfortable, ask for help. Mask fit, air leaks, dryness, pressure settings, nasal congestion, and sleeping position can often be adjusted or addressed.

Options may include airway-pressure therapy, a custom oral appliance, weight management, position changes, or surgery.

In the United States, tirzepatide (Zepbound), combined with a reduced-calorie diet and increased physical activity, is FDA-approved for moderate-to-severe OSA in adults with obesity. It is not right for everyone and does not replace follow-up to reassess sleep apnea or review the airway-pressure plan. Do not stop airway-pressure treatment solely because snoring improves.

SAFETY · SLEEPINESS AND DRIVING

Severe sleepiness can impair driving. If you are struggling to stay awake behind the wheel, do not drive. Arrange another way home and seek prompt medical evaluation.

Sleep can shape your blood pressure, rhythm, symptoms, and recovery. The next part turns from prevention to interpretation: what a new symptom, an unfamiliar diagnosis, a wearable alert, or a test result actually means.

FLOW PRACTICE · NOTICE THE NIGHT PATTERN

For one week, note whether you wake refreshed, have morning headaches or dry mouth, or are told you snore, gasp, or have pauses in breathing. Bring the pattern to your clinician; the notes cannot diagnose sleep apnea.

FLOW TAKEAWAY · CHAPTER 7

Sleep health includes duration, regularity, and breathing. OSA is more than snoring, and a sleep-study number should be interpreted with oxygen data, symptoms, study type, and other conditions. Treatment can improve breathing, alertness, quality of life, and blood pressure while the rest of the heart plan continues. If the pattern sounds familiar, ask whether sleep belongs in your next heart-care conversation.

PART III

Making Sense of Symptoms, Rhythm, and Tests

Interpretation

A symptom, label, alert, or test result is not the end of the reasoning. It is the beginning of the next question.

CHAPTER 8

When Flow Fails: Ischemia, Angina, and Heart Failure

Few words in cardiology sound as final as these three: ischemia, angina, heart failure. It is easy to hear them and assume your heart is broken, the damage is done, or your future has already been decided.

That is not what these words mean. They are related, but they are not interchangeable. When they blur together, the wrong worry attaches to the wrong problem. Separating them turns an alarming label back into information you can use.

SAFETY · IF THIS MIGHT BE AN EMERGENCY

If chest pressure, marked breathlessness, or another concerning symptom is new, worsening, severe, or occurs at rest, especially with sweating, fainting, nausea, confusion, or marked weakness, follow the Start Here guide and call emergency services. Do not drive yourself or use this chapter to decide whether a possible emergency can wait.

Ischemia: When Supply Cannot Meet Demand

Ischemia means oxygen supply to the heart muscle is not keeping up with demand. It is a state, not a picture on a scan. Causes include a plaque-related narrowing, temporary coronary spasm, abnormal regulation of the smallest coronary vessels, anemia, low blood oxygen or blood pressure, a rapid rhythm, or another stress that raises the heart's workload.

Ischemia can occur during exertion or at rest, and it may or may not cause angina. The word tells you that oxygen supply is falling short. It does not, by itself, tell you why, how severe the problem is, or how urgently it needs treatment. Cause, severity, timing, and duration provide that context.

Angina: The Symptom Pattern Ischemia Can Cause

Think of ischemia as what the heart muscle experiences. Angina is the chest discomfort ischemia can cause: pressure, squeezing, heaviness, or burning that may spread to the jaw, back, shoulder, or arm. Some people instead notice related symptoms, sometimes called ischemic equivalents, such as breathlessness or unusual fatigue.

Symptom quality alone cannot confirm or rule out a heart problem. Sharp pain is not an automatic all-clear, and a heart symptom does not have to feel dramatic. Clinicians use stable angina to describe a generally predictable pattern that eases with rest or prescribed medication. Symptoms that are new, worsening, provoked by less effort, or occurring at rest may signal an acute coronary syndrome, an urgent condition caused by suddenly reduced blood flow to the heart, and need immediate evaluation.

Reduced blood flow does not always announce itself. Silent ischemia is more common in people with diabetes, older adults, and people with nerve damage that affects automatic body functions, although it can occur in others. Risk factors alone cannot identify who has it, so routine screening is not appropriate for every person without symptoms.

Ischemia, Injury, Heart Attack, and Heart Failure

These terms often appear in the same conversation, but they describe different findings. Keeping them separate is what makes each one useful.

Table 8.1 · Five Labels That Are Not Interchangeable

TERM	MEANING AND BOUNDARY
Ischemia	**Means:** Oxygen supply does not meet the heart muscle's demand; it may be brief and reversible. **Does not mean:** Heart attack, permanent injury, or a major fixed blockage automatically.
Angina	**Means:** Chest discomfort caused by ischemia; breathlessness or fatigue may occur as ischemic equivalents. **Does not mean:** A fixed blockage has been proved. Ischemia can also occur without symptoms.
Myocardial injury	**Means:** A cardiac troponin blood test is above the laboratory's injury threshold. A rise or fall suggests recent injury; a persistently high level may reflect ongoing or chronic injury. **Does not mean:** The cause has been identified.
Heart attack (MI)	Means: Acute myocardial injury plus clinical evidence of acute ischemia. **Does not mean:** One elevated troponin value is enough by itself.
Heart failure	**Means:** A clinical syndrome in which a structural or functional heart abnormality causes symptoms or signs. **Does not mean:** The heart has stopped or the ejection fraction must be low.

Heart Failure Is Different

Heart failure can arise through more than one pathway. One person may have a heart that no longer squeezes strongly. Another may have a preserved ejection fraction yet fill only at abnormally high pressure. Valve disease, rhythm problems, heart-muscle disease, and other causes can produce the syndrome.

Heart failure can cause breathlessness, swelling, rapid fluid-related weight gain, fatigue, or declining exercise capacity. Those symptoms can also occur with lung disease, anemia, kidney disease, medication effects, or loss of fitness. They deserve clinical evaluation.

Ejection fraction, or EF, estimates the percentage of blood in the left ventricle that is pumped out with each beat. It is not a percentage score for the whole heart, and it is not the diagnosis.

Whatever the EF, symptoms alone do not establish heart failure. Clinicians also look for supporting evidence from the examination, echocardiogram, and sometimes blood tests called natriuretic peptides, which can rise when the heart is under strain. When EF is not clearly reduced, evidence of abnormal filling pressure or congestion becomes especially important.

Table 8.2 · What Ejection Fraction Can and Cannot Tell You

EF DESCRIPTION	WHAT IT CAN AND CANNOT TELL US
Reduced, 40% or lower	Squeezing strength is reduced. It does not establish the cause, symptom burden, reversibility, or complete treatment plan.
Mildly reduced, 41–49%	EF lies between the reduced and preserved ranges. The number alone does not establish heart failure or determine treatment.

EF DESCRIPTION	WHAT IT CAN AND CANNOT TELL US
Preserved, 50% or higher	The percentage ejected is not reduced. It does not exclude heart failure related to elevated filling pressure, valve disease, or another problem.
Improved, previously 40% or lower and now above 40%	EF has risen over time. It does not mean the underlying vulnerability has disappeared or treatment can safely stop.

Age, kidney disease, and atrial fibrillation can raise natriuretic-peptide levels, while obesity can lower them, so no single result should be read alone.

Heart failure can improve, remain stable, go into remission, or worsen. A low EF can lead to an effective treatment plan; it does not decide the future. Treatment has two jobs: relieve congestion and other symptoms, and address the cause and type of heart failure.

If your heart-failure team has given you a daily-weight, sodium, fluid, blood-pressure, or water-pill plan, follow that individualized plan rather than a general rule from this book.

Three Questions to Ask About Any Cardiac Label

When you receive one of these labels, ask three questions:

1. Is this describing a symptom, a test finding, or a diagnosis?
2. What evidence supports it, and what cause is suspected?
3. What decision or treatment changes because of it?

A label should guide the next step. It should not define your future.

FLOW TAKEAWAY · CHAPTER 8

Keep these labels separate. Ischemia is inadequate oxygen delivery for the heart's workload; angina is the chest discomfort it can cause. Myocardial injury, heart attack, and heart failure are different findings or diagnoses. Ask what evidence supports the label, what cause is suspected, and what treatment follows.

CHAPTER 9

Atrial Fibrillation: Rhythm, Stroke Risk, and Wearable Alerts

Your watch buzzes. On the screen: *possible atrial fibrillation.* For a moment, your own pulse seems to answer it, and a quiet evening becomes a question you do not know how urgently to take. Should you go to the emergency room? Ignore it? Call someone?

For many people, this is the first clue of a possible rhythm problem. The alert is not a diagnosis, but it deserves confirmation.

Much of this book is about coronary arteries, plaque, and blood flow. Atrial fibrillation begins in the heart's electrical system. It belongs in this story because it intersects with stroke, heart failure, blood pressure, sleep apnea, symptoms, and the decisions patients now face after a wearable alert.

Normally, the upper chambers of the heart, called the atria, contract in an organized way before the lower chambers pump. In atrial fibrillation, or AFib, electrical activity in the atria becomes chaotic. The atria quiver instead of squeezing normally. The pulse is irregular and may be fast, and the rhythm may come and go or become continuous.

Atrial Fibrillation: Three Things to Understand

AFib changes the heart's electrical rhythm. It also creates two separate care decisions.

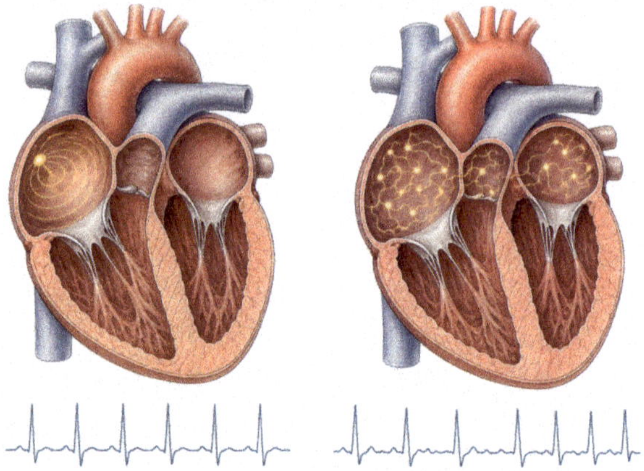

NORMAL RHYTHM

One organized signal starts each heartbeat.

ATRIAL FIBRILLATION

Signals become disorganized; the atria quiver and the pulse is irregular.

Stroke prevention

AFib can allow blood to pool and a clot to form. The anticoagulant decision depends on stroke risk, bleeding risk, and preferences.

Rate, rhythm, and symptoms

Rate control, rhythm treatment, or a procedure may help. The plan depends on symptoms, AFib duration, other conditions, and goals.

A wearable alert is a clue, not a diagnosis.
A clinician confirms AFib on an ECG-quality tracing.

Figure 9.1 · What Atrial Fibrillation Changes. AFib disrupts electrical activity in the atria and usually makes the pulse irregular. Care then follows two separate tracks: reducing stroke risk and managing rate, rhythm, and symptoms. Confirmation requires clinician review of an electrocardiogram (ECG)-quality tracing.

When a Watch Sends an Alert

A wearable can generate two different kinds of information. A pulse-irregularity notification uses light sensors to flag a pattern that might be AFib. Motion, poor skin contact, premature beats, and other rhythms can produce a similar alert. A single-lead electrocardiogram (ECG) records an electrical signal and may provide stronger evidence, but the tracing still needs visual review by a qualified clinician. A pulse alert alone is not enough to diagnose AFib.

If you feel well and receive an isolated alert, it usually calls for clinician follow-up, not an automatic trip to the emergency department. Save the tracing or screenshot if the device recorded one. Note the time, your symptoms and activity, and anything unusual such as illness, dehydration, poor sleep, or alcohol. Repeated alerts or sustained symptoms deserve more prompt attention.

SAFETY · WHEN AN IRREGULAR RHYTHM IS AN EMERGENCY

Call 911 for signs of stroke, including new facial droop, arm weakness, trouble speaking, or sudden loss of balance or vision. Also call for severe chest pressure, fainting, severe breathlessness, confusion, profound weakness, or a very low blood-pressure reading with symptoms. Do not drive yourself.

Once AFib is confirmed, care follows two related but separate tracks. How you feel is not the same as your stroke risk. A person with dramatic palpitations may have a low risk of stroke, while someone who feels normal may still need stroke prevention. Clinicians therefore ask two questions separately: How should stroke risk be reduced, and how should the rhythm be managed?

Track One: Preventing Stroke

When the atria quiver instead of squeezing effectively, blood stagnates, and can form a clot, particularly in a pouch called the left atrial appendage. A clot that leaves the heart can travel to the brain and cause a stroke.

Stroke risk is not determined by how strongly you feel AFib or whether it occurs every day. Clinicians estimate risk using factors such as age, high blood pressure, diabetes, heart failure, prior stroke, and vascular disease. That assessment guides the decision about an anticoagulant, a medicine that reduces the blood's tendency to form harmful clots.

For most people with AFib who need anticoagulation, a direct oral anticoagulant is preferred over warfarin. Warfarin is generally used instead for a mechanical heart valve or moderate-to-severe narrowing of the mitral valve caused by rheumatic disease. Aspirin is not an adequate substitute for anticoagulation in AFib.

Anticoagulants lower stroke risk but can increase bleeding. The plan should account for kidney function, other medicines, prior bleeding, fall risk, and personal preferences. A tendency to fall should prompt fall-prevention and bleeding-safety planning. It should not automatically rule out anticoagulation when benefit is likely.

Do not stop an anticoagulant because the pulse feels normal or a watch no longer detects AFib.

After ablation, current guidelines still base long-term anticoagulation mainly on stroke risk rather than whether the rhythm seems normal. New trials suggest that some carefully selected patients without documented recurrence for at least a year may be able to stop under specialist supervision, but the evidence is still evolving. Never stop an anticoagulant on your own.

For selected patients who cannot safely take long-term anticoagulation, or who face an unusually high risk of major bleeding, a procedure to close the left atrial appendage may be considered. It is not a routine or automatically safer alternative.

Track Two: Rate or Rhythm

Rate control allows AFib to continue while slowing the lower chambers so the heart is not racing. Rhythm control tries to restore and maintain a normal rhythm with medicine, cardioversion (an electrical reset), ablation (a catheter procedure that blocks abnormal electrical signals), or a combination.

For some people with recently diagnosed AFib and additional cardiovascular risk, early rhythm control can improve cardiovascular outcomes. I frame the choice around the goal: relief of symptoms, better heart function, slower AFib progression, or fewer cardiovascular events. The strategy also depends on how long AFib has been present, other conditions, procedural risk, and the patient's priorities. Stroke prevention remains a separate decision even when normal rhythm is restored.

EVIDENCE SNAPSHOT 9.1

Why Early Rhythm Control Deserves Discussion

EAST-AFNET 4 · NEW ENGLAND JOURNAL OF MEDICINE, 2020

WHAT WAS STUDIED

EAST-AFNET 4 assigned 2,789 people whose AFib had been diagnosed within the previous year and who had additional cardiovascular conditions to early rhythm control or usual care.

WHAT RESEARCHERS FOUND

Over a median of 5.1 years, the main combined outcome occurred at 3.9 versus 5.0 events per 100 person-years. It included cardiovascular death, stroke, or hospitalization for worsening heart failure or an acute coronary syndrome.

WHAT THIS MEANS

Early rhythm control deserves discussion for selected patients soon after diagnosis.

IMPORTANT LIMIT

This was a treatment-strategy trial, not an ablation-only trial; rhythm control included medicines, cardioversion, ablation, or a combination. Restoring normal rhythm does not automatically remove the need for stroke prevention.

For Readers Who Want the Deeper Layer: Short Device-Detected Episodes

An implanted pacemaker or defibrillator can record brief atrial high-rate episodes before clinical AFib appears on a standard ECG. These episodes are not the same as a consumer-watch alert. The anticoagulation decision depends on episode duration and the person's stroke and bleeding risks.

EVIDENCE SNAPSHOT 9.2

When an Implanted Device Finds Brief Atrial Episodes

ARTESiA AND NOAH-AFNET 6 · NEW ENGLAND JOURNAL OF MEDICINE, 2023–2024

WHAT WAS STUDIED

ARTESiA and NOAH-AFNET 6 studied people with atrial episodes detected by implanted devices but no ECG-documented clinical AFib.

WHAT RESEARCHERS FOUND

In ARTESiA, the annual rate of stroke or systemic embolism, a clot blocking an artery elsewhere in the body, fell from 1.24% with aspirin to 0.78% with apixaban, while major bleeding rose from 0.94% to 1.71%. In NOAH-AFNET 6, edoxaban did not significantly reduce cardiovascular death, stroke, or systemic embolism and increased death or major bleeding.

WHAT THIS MEANS

Anticoagulation is not automatic. Episode duration and the individual risks of stroke and bleeding matter.

IMPORTANT LIMIT

The trials used different medicines, comparison groups, and outcomes. Neither result applies directly to a consumer-watch alert.

Not Every Racing Heart Is AFib

Palpitations have many causes. Extra beats can feel like skips or thumps. A fast rhythm that begins above the heart's lower chambers, called supraventricular tachycardia, often feels rapid but regular. Fever, anxiety, anemia, dehydration, thyroid disease, stimulants, and exercise can all increase a normal heart rate.

Postural orthostatic tachycardia syndrome, or POTS, is not AFib. It involves an excessive rise in heart rate with standing and has a different mechanism and treatment. Recording the rhythm helps distinguish these conditions.

Blood-pressure control, regular activity, weight reduction when appropriate, and limiting or avoiding alcohol can reduce AFib episodes or recurrence in some people. Because sleep-disordered breathing is common in AFib, screening may be appropriate. Treatment can improve sleep-related health, although whether it reliably reduces AFib burden remains uncertain. These steps do not replace an anticoagulant when stroke risk calls for one.

FLOW PRACTICE · MAKE THE TWO-TRACK PLAN

At your next AFib visit, divide a page into two headings: Stroke protection and Rate/rhythm. Before you leave, know what the plan is under each.

FLOW TAKEAWAY · CHAPTER 9

AFib creates two tracks: protect the brain from stroke and decide how to manage rate or rhythm. Save a wearable tracing for review; a clinician still needs to confirm the rhythm. Even after cardioversion or ablation, stroke risk gets its own decision.

Use next: Flow Tool 14, If Your Watch Flags Possible AFib.

CHAPTER 10

What a "Normal" Test Actually Means

"Your test is normal" can be exactly the reassurance a patient needs. It can also be misunderstood. Earlier, I told you about a man in his fifties whose stress test had been reassuring. I return to him here because he changed how I say that sentence.

When chest pressure began one evening, he almost stayed home. He believed his heart had already been checked.

He was not my patient until that night. I was the cardiologist on call when he arrived in the middle of a large heart attack, his blood pressure already failing. We opened the artery and placed a temporary heart pump to support his circulation. He reached the intensive care unit, but the injury was too extensive. He died the next day.

What I remember most is his family's bewilderment. Not anger, but bewilderment. The earlier test had found no evidence that blood supply fell short under the conditions tested. It had not mapped every plaque or predicted which one might later change and trigger a clot.

The test had not lied. It had answered the question it was built to answer. What failed was the promise everyone had heard in the word *normal.*

FLOW TRUTH

A new symptom creates a new question. Severe, worsening, or resting symptoms deserve fresh assessment even after a reassuring test.

A Test Changes Probability

Before ordering a test, a clinician estimates how likely a condition is based on the symptoms, timing, examination, age, risk factors, and previous results. The test moves that estimate up or down. It rarely turns it into zero or 100 percent.

A negative result is most reassuring when the right test was chosen, the study was completed well, and the chance of disease was not already very high. It is less reassuring when symptoms are strongly concerning, the study was limited, or the test did not assess the suspected problem well.

The reverse matters too. When a condition was very unlikely before testing, an unexpected abnormality is more likely to be a false-positive result (a finding that looks abnormal even though the condition is not present) and may need confirmation before it drives treatment.

A useful interpretation answers three questions:

1. How likely was the condition before the test?
2. How much did the result change that estimate?
3. What decision changes now?

Why Normal Results Can Feel So Wrong

A normal result often becomes a stopping point. That is reasonable only when it closes the question that mattered. If symptoms persist, reopen both cardiac and noncardiac possibilities. Do not let either anxiety or microvascular disease become a shortcut diagnosis.

On a report, "normal" may mean no major blockage, no ischemia under the conditions tested, or reassuring heart structure and function. Name the finding precisely. Then add the safety instruction: new, worsening, severe, or resting symptoms require a new assessment.

Why Doctors Sometimes Sound Uncertain

I sometimes have to tell a patient, "I'm not sure yet." When the evidence is incomplete, that is the most accurate answer I can give. The next conversation should make the uncertainty useful: Which causes still fit? How confident are we in the current explanation? What finding would change the plan?

Normal, Negative, or Nondiagnostic?

Reports sometimes use these words loosely, but the distinction is useful.

- A **normal** result means the measured findings fell within the expected range.
- A **negative** result means the test did not find the condition it was designed to detect.
- A nondiagnostic or inconclusive result means the study could not answer the question with enough confidence.

A stress study may be limited if the person cannot exercise hard enough, the images are unclear, motion or an irregular rhythm distorts the signal, or the heart does not reach the intended level of stress. Ask, "Was the study technically adequate and diagnostic for the question we were asking?"

When a Normal Result Really Is Reassuring

I am usually comfortable pausing cardiac testing when the right test was completed well, symptoms have resolved or remain stable without warning signs, and the chance of dangerous disease is low. More testing at that moment is unlikely to help. The patient should leave knowing the follow-up plan and which changes would reopen the question.

When symptoms continue, the next step is not automatically more of the same testing. It is asking which plausible cause the first test did not examine.

FLOW PRACTICE · ASK "NORMAL FOR WHAT?"

Before you file away a "normal" report, write down what the test assessed, whether it was technically adequate, and which changes should reopen the question.

FLOW TAKEAWAY · CHAPTER 10

After a "normal" result, ask what the test assessed, whether it was technically adequate, and which symptoms or changes should bring you back.

Use next: Flow Tool 4, Questions After a Normal Stress Test.

CHAPTER 11

When Symptoms Persist After Reassuring Tests

The woman from Chapter 5 eventually had the measurement her earlier tests had not provided: her coronary blood flow could not rise normally under stress. That supported dysfunction in the heart's smallest vessels. Her symptoms were real, but the diagnosis did not come from symptoms alone.

That distinction matters. If your symptoms persist after reassuring tests, the next step is not to assume microvascular disease, spasm, anxiety, or any other single cause. It is to ask what the earlier tests did and did not assess, then look for evidence that can separate the possibilities.

You can follow the rest of this chapter without remembering these acronyms.

OPTIONAL · FOR READERS WHO WANT THE TERMS

Table 11.1 · Terms You May See After Reassuring Tests

Term	Plain-language meaning
ANOCA	Symptoms consistent with angina, but no major coronary blockage is found. It describes the clinical pattern, not the cause.

Term	Plain-language meaning
INOCA	Testing shows that the heart muscle is not receiving enough oxygen-rich blood for its workload, but no major blockage explains it. Small-vessel dysfunction or spasm may be responsible.
MINOCA	A heart attack is confirmed, but angiography finds no major blockage to explain it. This acute working diagnosis still requires a search for the cause.
Coronary microvascular dysfunction	The heart's small vessels do not regulate blood flow normally. It can cause ANOCA or INOCA and can coexist with large-artery disease or spasm.

When a Reassuring Test Does Not Explain the Symptoms

Reopen the possibilities: coronary spasm, a rhythm disorder, lung disease, anemia, digestive or musculoskeletal causes, medication effects, anxiety or panic, and other explanations. Rank them by the symptom pattern and the testing already completed. Neither microvascular disease nor anxiety should become a default answer.

When confirmed, coronary microvascular dysfunction can explain angina or ischemia without a flow-limiting blockage in a major artery. Some objectively measured forms are associated with impaired quality of life and higher cardiovascular risk. Treatment is individualized and often combines risk-factor control, symptom-directed medicines, activity or rehabilitation, and follow-up.

Coronary Spasm Is a Different Mechanism

Coronary spasm is a temporary abnormal constriction. It may involve a large surface artery (epicardial spasm) or smaller coronary vessels (microvascular spasm). Epicardial spasm can produce chest pressure and ischemic ECG changes and, rarely, a heart attack even though the artery looks open between episodes.

Spasm requires a different treatment strategy from impaired small-vessel dilation. That is why identifying the likely mechanism matters.

How Microvascular Function and Spasm Are Assessed

A routine angiogram does not directly test small-vessel function or coronary spasm.

Optional: How Coronary Function Is Tested

Positron emission tomography (PET) blood-flow imaging and stress cardiac magnetic resonance imaging (MRI) can assess how blood reaches the heart muscle and, at expert centers, measure blood flow or flow reserve. These tests can support a diagnosis of impaired microvascular function, but they do not test every mechanism or provoke coronary spasm.

In a specialized catheterization laboratory, clinicians can measure coronary flow reserve (how much blood flow can increase) and microvascular resistance (how much resistance the smallest vessels create). They may also give acetylcholine, a medicine that can provoke spasm under monitored conditions, to test for large-artery or small-vessel spasm. These tests are used selectively when the result is likely to change treatment.

FLOW TRUTH

A routine angiogram can rule out a major obstructive lesion. It does not measure coronary flow reserve or test for spasm, and neither diagnosis should be assigned from symptoms alone.

When atherosclerosis or vascular risk is present, prevention still matters. Symptom treatment is matched to the suspected or measured mechanism. So far, the evidence is stronger for improving symptoms and quality of life than for preventing a heart attack or death.

EVIDENCE SNAPSHOT 11.1

Coronary Function Testing Matched to Treatment

CorMicA · JOURNAL OF THE AMERICAN COLLEGE OF CARDIOLOGY, 2018; JACC: CARDIOVASCULAR INTERVENTIONS, 2020

WHAT WAS STUDIED

In a randomized trial, 151 people with angina and no obstructive coronary artery disease underwent invasive coronary-function testing. In the intervention group, results were disclosed and used to guide treatment; the comparison group received usual care while the results remained blinded.

WHAT RESEARCHERS FOUND

Mechanism-guided care improved angina and quality of life at six months, and the benefit was sustained at one year.

WHAT THIS MEANS

Mechanism-guided care can improve symptoms in selected patients.

IMPORTANT LIMIT

This modest trial was conducted at two centers in one health system and was not powered to show fewer heart attacks or deaths. Major cardiovascular events were similar between groups.

Treatment Follows the Mechanism

When testing suggests that the small vessels cannot widen enough, treatment addresses vascular risk and coexisting disease. Options for symptoms may include a beta blocker, ranolazine, a calcium-channel blocker, rehabilitation, or another strategy. The choice depends on heart rate, blood pressure, symptoms, other conditions, and response.

For epicardial or microvascular spasm confirmed during testing, calcium-channel blockers are generally first-line treatment. Nitrates may help, particularly with epicardial vasospasm. Some beta blockers, especially nonselective ones, can aggravate vasospasm, so do not stop or change one without guidance.

More than one mechanism can be present. Reassess whether episodes are less frequent, daily activity is easier, or side effects have created a new problem. If the response does not fit, revisit the diagnosis before simply increasing the same medicine. Once the possibilities are narrowed, ask whether another test could distinguish them well enough to change care.

FLOW PRACTICE · CAPTURE THE PATTERN

For non-emergency symptoms, record what you were doing, how long they lasted, what relieved them, and any wearable reading. New, severe, or worsening symptoms still require prompt care.

FLOW TAKEAWAY · CHAPTER 11

When symptoms persist after large-vessel testing, keep cardiac and noncardiac causes in view. Test microvascular function or spasm selectively, then match treatment to the mechanism supported by evidence. If symptoms continue, ask which plausible cause the testing did not examine before repeating more of the same.
Use next: Flow Tool 11, Symptom and Trend Tracker, and the FLOWS Symptom-Description Aid.

CHAPTER 12

Matching the Test to the Question

A test should earn its place by answering a question that is still open. Before I order one, I ask what the earlier studies have already settled, what they could not assess, and what I would do differently with a positive, negative, or uncertain result.

This chapter organizes the common tests by the job each one does: detecting acute injury, showing plaque, assessing structure, measuring blood flow under stress, or finding a risk we can treat. Some abbreviations appear in the overview: FFR and iFR are pressure measurements across a narrowing, while PET and cardiac MRI are scans that can assess blood flow to heart muscle. A useful result changes treatment, follow-up, or reassurance. Otherwise, testing can add noise.

What Each Cardiac Test Can Tell You

TEST	WHAT IT CAN TELL YOU
ECG / EKG	Rhythm and electrical activity; may show ischemic changes or prior injury.
Serial troponin	Heart-muscle injury and its rise-or-fall pattern; not the cause by itself.
Echocardiogram	Pumping, filling, valves, wall motion, and other structure; not coronary plaque.
Calcium score (CAC)	Calcified coronary plaque burden; not noncalcified plaque, ischemia, or an acute syndrome.
Coronary CT angiography (CCTA)	Plaque location, type, and narrowing; not whether every narrowing limits flow.
Stress test	The heart's response to exercise or medication stress; the signal depends on the method.
Invasive coronary angiography	The contrast-filled channel in larger coronary arteries; not all wall plaque or microvascular function.
FFR / iFR	Whether a specific narrowing is likely to limit blood flow enough to matter.
PET / CMR / flow reserve	Blood flow to the heart muscle or flow reserve in selected patients; methods and availability vary.

A "normal" result answers only the question the test was designed to ask.

Figure 12.1 · What Each Cardiac Test Can Tell You. The same word, "normal," means something different on an ECG, a troponin test, an echocardiogram, a stress test, a plaque-imaging study, or a pressure measurement.

Is There Acute Injury or an Electrical Emergency?

An electrocardiogram (ECG) records the heart's electrical activity. It can show changes associated with reduced blood flow, rhythm disturbances, conduction problems, or prior injury. A normal ECG does not, by itself, exclude a heart attack.

Troponin signals heart-muscle injury, not its cause. Clinicians often repeat it to see whether the level is rising or falling. The result is interpreted with symptoms, ECG findings, timing, and the assay used; a single value obtained too early does not always settle the question.

Is Calcified Coronary Plaque Present, and How Much?

Coronary artery calcium, or CAC, scoring is mainly a preventive risk tool for people without active symptoms. In selected low-risk patients with stable chest pain, it is also an option as a first-line test for calcified plaque. It cannot rule out an acute coronary syndrome, meaning an urgent problem caused by suddenly reduced blood flow to the heart, or detect noncalcified plaque or whether blood supply is falling short. It must not be used to self-triage new, worsening, severe, or resting symptoms.

- **Zero:** No calcified plaque is detected, and near-term risk is generally lower. Noncalcified plaque and other causes of symptoms can still be present.
- **1–99:** Calcified plaque is present. Age and how the score compares with others of similar age and sex help place it in context.
- **100–399:** Plaque burden is greater and risk is higher, often supporting more intensive prevention.

- **400 and above:** Calcified plaque burden is extensive and risk is high. The need for angiography or a stent still depends on symptoms and evidence of flow limitation.

A calcium score does not predict a specific event, but it can reveal hidden risk early enough to change prevention.

How Is the Heart Structured and Functioning?

Echocardiography assesses chamber size, pumping and filling, wall motion, valves, estimated pressures, and the sac around the heart. It does not show plaque in the coronary arteries.

What Do CCTA and Invasive Angiography Show?

Coronary CT angiography, or CCTA, shows the location and extent of plaque, classifies it as calcified, noncalcified, or mixed, and estimates how much it narrows the open channel. Certain CT features are associated with higher risk across groups, but a scan cannot identify which plaque, if any, will later cause an event. CCTA maps the present; it cannot forecast a specific plaque's future.

Invasive coronary angiography, performed during cardiac catheterization, uses a thin tube inserted through an artery at the wrist or groin and contrast dye to outline the open channel inside the larger coronary arteries. The same procedure can allow pressure measurements or treatment when indicated.

Coronary calcium scoring and CCTA answer different questions. Calcium scoring usually refines preventive risk; CCTA maps plaque and narrowing when symptoms or another anatomic question warrants a closer look. Most people need the study matched to the question, not both.

FLOW TRUTH

Invaseness and completeness are different. Each test provides a different view.

Three Tests, Three Different Views

Each test answers a different question.

CORONARY CTA

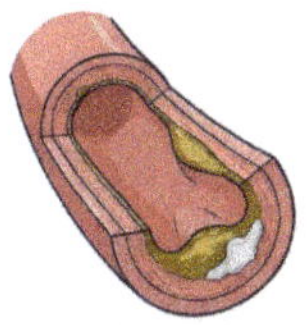

Maps plaque in the artery wall

Shows calcified and noncalcified plaque and estimates narrowing.

Limit: It does not prove whether a narrowing limits blood flow.

STRESS TESTING

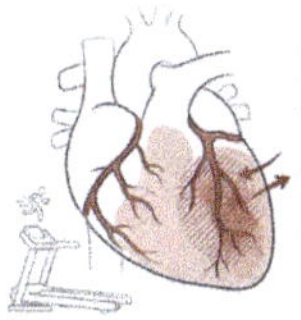

Assesses blood supply under stress

Looks for signs that blood supply falls short under stress.

Limit: It does not map plaque in the artery wall.

INVASIVE ANGIOGRAPHY

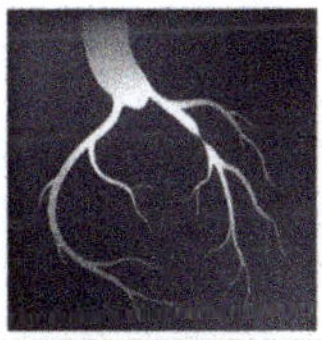

Outlines the open channel

Shows the contrast-filled channel. Pressure can be measured or treatment performed when indicated.

Limit: It does not show all plaque within the artery wall.

CCTA maps plaque. Stress testing assesses blood supply under stress. Invasive angiography outlines the open channel.

The best test depends on the question. No single view answers every question.

Figure 12.2 · Three Tests, Three Different Views. CCTA maps plaque; stress testing assesses blood supply under stress; invasive angiography outlines the open channel and can permit pressure measurement or treatment.

Does Blood Supply Fall Short Under Stress?

Stress tests use exercise or medication to change cardiac demand or coronary blood flow. Each method looks for a different signal.

During angiography, fractional flow reserve (FFR) and instantaneous wave-free ratio (iFR) use pressure measurements across a specific narrowing to estimate whether it is likely to limit blood flow enough to matter. Positron emission tomography (PET) blood-flow imaging and stress cardiac magnetic resonance imaging (MRI) can show how blood reaches the heart muscle. In selected patients, these and other flow-reserve tests can support evaluation of small-vessel dysfunction.

Five Common Stress-Test Methods

Exercise ECG

MAIN SIGNAL Symptoms, exercise capacity, heart rate, blood pressure, and ECG changes during exercise.

USEFUL FEATURES AND LIMITS
Provides useful functional information without imaging. It is less useful when the resting ECG cannot be read for ischemia or the patient cannot exercise adequately.

Stress Echocardiography

MAIN SIGNAL Heart-muscle contraction and valve or pressure findings during exercise or medication stress.

USEFUL FEATURES AND LIMITS
Avoids radiation and adds structural information. Image quality and reader expertise matter.

Single-Photon Emission Computed Tomography (SPECT)

MAIN SIGNAL How a small amount of tracer distributes through the heart muscle during stress and rest.

USEFUL FEATURES AND LIMITS
Widely available. Radiation, soft-tissue shadows, and the fact that images compare one area with another can affect interpretation.

PET Blood-Flow Imaging

MAIN SIGNAL Blood flow to the heart muscle and, at many centers, how much flow can increase.

USEFUL FEATURES AND LIMITS
Offers strong image quality and can help assess small-vessel function. Availability is limited, and methods vary.

Stress Cardiac MRI

MAIN SIGNAL Blood flow, wall motion, pumping function, and features of the heart muscle during medication stress.

USEFUL FEATURES AND LIMITS
Avoids ionizing radiation and provides detailed muscle information. It may not suit some implants or devices, severe claustrophobia, or certain kidney-related contrast concerns.

When a patient tells me a stress test was "normal," I ask which kind. A normal exercise ECG, SPECT image, PET flow measurement, and stress MRI do not mean exactly the same thing. The report should say what signal was measured and whether exercise or image quality limited the answer.

When I choose among stress tests, I first ask whether the patient can exercise and whether the resting ECG is interpretable.

Then I consider kidney function, contrast allergy, radiation, rhythm, earlier tests, expected image quality, and local expertise. The best study is the one that can answer the clinical question well enough to guide the next step.

Which Risks Can Be Treated?

Blood tests answer other questions. A lipid panel and glucose or A1c identify treatable risk. ApoB estimates the number of plaque-forming particles and can help when LDL cholesterol and particle number disagree. Lp(a), an inherited risk factor, should generally be measured at least once in adulthood.

Other tests are selected for the clinical question. High-sensitivity C-reactive protein (hs-CRP), a general inflammation marker, can add information in some situations but does not identify where inflammation comes from. A blood count can identify anemia. Thyroid testing can help explain some rhythm or cholesterol problems. Kidney function, liver enzymes, sodium, and potassium can guide medicine choice and monitoring.

One test shows plaque. Another shows whether blood supply falls short under stress. An echocardiogram shows how the heart is working, and blood tests identify risks that can be treated. Read together, the results become a clinical picture rather than a stack of reports.

BEFORE THE NEXT TEST

Ask three questions: What will this test answer? What can it miss? What would a positive, negative, or uncertain result lead us to do differently?

Once the right question meets the right test, you still need to know what the answer changes: medicine, a procedure, follow-up, or reassurance. A finding is information. It does not make the decision by itself.

FLOW TAKEAWAY · CHAPTER 12

Start with the unanswered question, not the next available scan. Ask what each possible result would lead you and your clinician to do differently.

Use next: Flow Tool 9, Questions Before a Planned Test or Procedure.

PART IV

Procedures and Medicines

Intervention

Begin by naming the job: restore blood flow, relieve symptoms, or reduce risk over time.

CHAPTER 13

Stents and Bypass: When Procedures Save Lives and When Their Job Is Different

When a test shows a narrowing in one of your coronary arteries, a stent can feel like the obvious answer: a blockage was found, so the blockage should be fixed. Sometimes that is exactly right. I have watched an emergency stent reopen a suddenly closed artery and save threatened heart muscle within minutes.

In stable disease, the same device usually has a different job: relieving symptoms. A stent treats one site. Medicines and risk-factor treatment protect the vascular system beyond the single place a stent can reach. Before recommending any planned procedure, I ask one question: **What outcome are we trying to change?**

During percutaneous coronary intervention (PCI), a cardiologist advances a thin tube from the wrist or groin to the heart. A wire crosses the narrowing, a balloon opens it, and a mesh stent holds that spot open. Bypass surgery uses an artery or vein graft to route blood around one or more narrowings.

When Restoring Blood Flow Urgently Can Save Heart Muscle and Life

Restoring blood flow is called revascularization. An ST-elevation myocardial infarction (STEMI) is a heart attack with an electrocardiogram (ECG) pattern that often points to a fully blocked artery. Treatment usually means emergency catheterization and PCI when appropriate. Other heart attacks may also require urgent catheterization for persistent symptoms, unstable circulation, or a dangerous rhythm.

In those moments, the goal is immediate: restore flow before more heart muscle is permanently injured. I still remember a middle-of-the-night case in which the monitor changed as the wire crossed and the artery opened: the rhythm steadied, the pressure improved, and the room changed with it. That is what emergency PCI is built to do.

Treatment during a heart attack usually begins with the artery causing the event. Other important narrowings may also need attention, but not always during the same procedure. Their timing depends on the patient's stability, kidney function, and the location and complexity of the disease. A narrowing that is not causing the emergency should be judged on its own rather than treated automatically.

The left main coronary artery is a short vessel that supplies a large amount of heart muscle. When the left main or several major arteries are significantly diseased, a Heart Team (typically including an interventional cardiologist, a cardiac surgeon, and other specialists as needed) should compare PCI with bypass surgery. The discussion should include durability, recovery, procedural risk, diabetes, heart function, and what matters most to the patient.

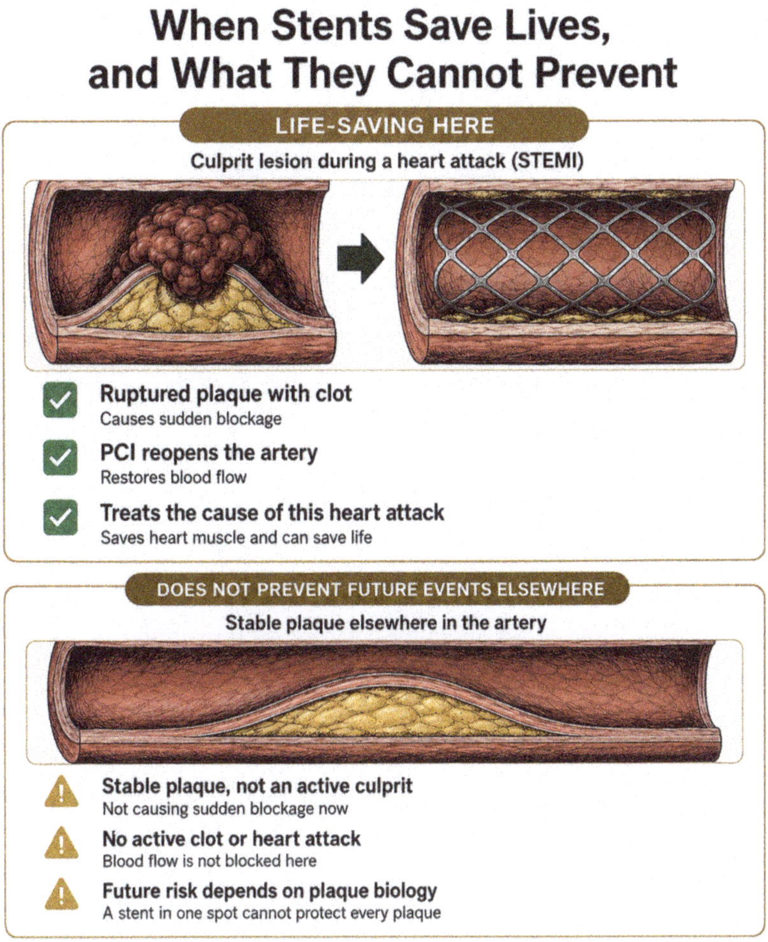

Figure 13.1 · When Stents Save Lives, and What They Cannot Prevent. During a heart attack, PCI can reopen the culprit artery and save heart muscle. A stent treats one site; medicines and risk-factor treatment address plaque throughout the vascular system.

When Stents Mainly Improve Symptoms

With stable, predictable chest discomfort, PCI can reduce angina and improve quality of life when a specific narrowing explains symptoms that continue despite medical therapy. Symptom relief is not a lesser outcome. When angina limits walking, work, exercise, or daily life, better function can justify a planned procedure even when it is not expected to prolong life.

Benefit is greatest when symptoms are frequent or limiting. A person with little or no angina should not expect the same improvement.

For many patients with stable coronary disease, routinely starting with angiography and a possible procedure has not reduced death or heart attack compared with guideline-based medicines and risk-factor treatment. That answers an important survival question. It does not erase the separate question of symptoms and quality of life.

A procedure may still be appropriate when symptoms continue despite treatment, when disease has a high-risk pattern, or when other findings change the goal.

EVIDENCE SNAPSHOT 13.1

What Procedures Change in Stable Coronary Disease

COURAGE AND ISCHEMIA · NEW ENGLAND JOURNAL OF MEDICINE, 2007 AND 2020

WHAT WAS STUDIED

Two major trials asked whether routinely starting with angiography and a possible procedure changes survival or heart-attack risk compared with guideline-based medicines and risk-factor treatment.

TRIAL	WHAT RESEARCHERS FOUND
COURAGE	Adding PCI did not reduce death or heart attack. PCI relieved angina sooner, although the difference narrowed over time.
ISCHEMIA	A routine invasive start did not reduce death or heart attack overall. People with angina—especially frequent angina—had greater improvement in symptoms and quality of life.

WHAT THIS MEANS

In stable disease, a procedure can offer meaningful symptom relief even when it is not expected to prolong life.

IMPORTANT LIMIT

These findings do not apply to an active heart attack, unstable symptoms, significant left-main disease, or every high-risk pattern of coronary disease.

Medical Therapy, PCI, and Bypass Do Different Jobs

Medicines and Risk-Factor Treatment

This is the foundation of chronic coronary care, whether or not a procedure is performed. It lowers risk throughout the vascular system and can reduce angina. It requires consistent use, follow-up, and adjustment, and symptoms may remain despite treatment.

PCI With a Stent

PCI restores blood flow at one specific narrowing and usually has a shorter recovery than surgery. It is used in emergencies and for persistent symptoms linked to a treatable narrowing. Antiplatelet medicines, which make platelets less likely to form a clot, are essential afterward.

Coronary Bypass Surgery

Bypass creates new routes around several narrowed arteries. It is major surgery with a longer recovery. It is often considered for significant left-main disease, complex disease in several arteries, selected patients with diabetes, or anatomy less suited to PCI.

These are not competing slogans. They are layers of care. Revascularization addresses a defined flow problem; long-term therapy reduces risk across the vascular system.

The Role of FFR and iFR

An angiogram shows what the dye-filled artery looks like. Fractional flow reserve (FFR) or instantaneous wave-free ratio (iFR) estimates what a particular narrowing does to blood flow. That distinction can change the decision: a narrowing that looks important may have little effect on flow, while another may be confirmed as flow-limiting.

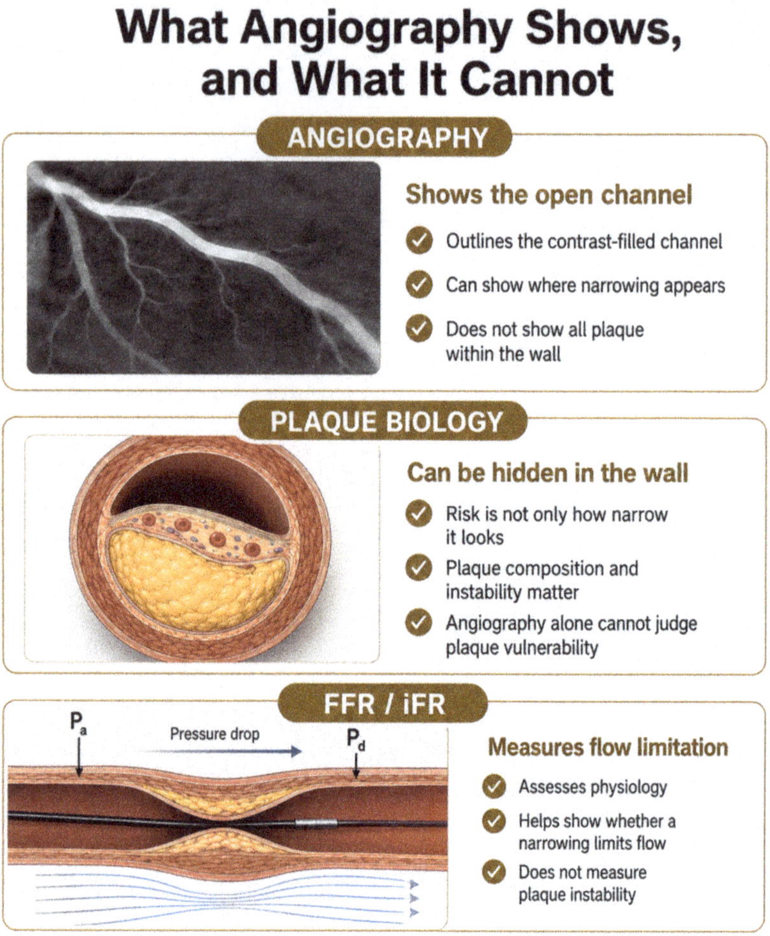

Figure 13.2 · What Angiography Shows, and What It Cannot. Angiography outlines the contrast-filled channel. FFR and iFR assess whether a narrowing limits flow. Neither directly shows plaque biology or vulnerability.

EVIDENCE SNAPSHOT 13.2

When a Pressure Measurement Supports PCI

FAME 2 AND FIVE-YEAR FOLLOW-UP · NEW ENGLAND JOURNAL OF MEDICINE, 2012 AND 2018

WHAT WAS STUDIED

FAME 2 randomized 888 people with stable coronary disease and at least one narrowing with an FFR of 0.80 or lower to FFR-guided PCI plus medical therapy or medical therapy alone.

WHAT RESEARCHERS FOUND

Over five years, the combined outcome of death, heart attack, or urgent revascularization occurred in 13.9% with PCI plus medical therapy and 27.0% with medical therapy alone. The difference was driven mainly by fewer urgent procedures. Death and heart attack were not significantly different when examined separately.

PRESSURE RESULT	HOW IT MAY INFORM CARE
FFR ≤ 0.80	Abnormal; may support PCI in a selected patient.
FFR > 0.80	PCI can often be deferred when the rest of the clinical picture fits.

WHAT THIS MEANS

A pressure measurement can support the decision; it does not make the decision by itself.

IMPORTANT LIMIT
An abnormal FFR does not automatically require a stent. Symptoms, anatomy, heart function, overall risk, and patient preferences still matter.

Procedure Risks and the Antiplatelet Plan

PCI can cause bleeding or blood-vessel injury where the catheter entered. Contrast dye can cause an allergic reaction or kidney injury in susceptible patients. The procedure can also damage a coronary artery. Heart attack, stroke, emergency surgery, and death are uncommon but possible.

Risk is not the same for every patient. It changes with the urgency of the procedure, the pattern of coronary disease, kidney function, anemia, vascular disease, frailty, and other illnesses. Bypass surgery has a different risk profile and a longer recovery because it is major surgery.

CRITICAL SAFETY RULE

After a recent stent, do not stop any prescribed antiplatelet medicine without explicit instructions from the cardiology team. For dental work, planned surgery, side effects, or non-emergency bleeding, contact the cardiology team before interrupting treatment. Call 911 for severe bleeding or another emergency.

EVIDENCE IN CONTEXT 13.3

Can Selected High-Risk Plaques Be Treated Before They Limit Flow?

PROSPECT ABSORB first tested this idea in 182 patients after a heart attack who had non-flow-limiting plaques with a large plaque burden. PCI enlarged the lumen, but the pilot was designed around an imaging outcome and did not establish fewer heart attacks or deaths.

PREVENT then studied 1,606 patients with a non-flow-limiting plaque and specific high-risk features on imaging from inside the artery. At two years, the primary combined outcome occurred in 0.4% with preventive PCI and 3.4% with medical therapy alone. The difference largely reflected fewer later hospitalizations and repeat procedures; death and heart attack were not clearly lower when examined separately.

This is an active research question in a narrowly selected setting. It does not support searching for or stenting every non-flow-limiting plaque, and preventive PCI is not routine care.

SOURCE PROSPECT ABSORB, JACC, 2020; PREVENT, The Lancet, 2024.

Questions to Ask Before Any Planned Stent

- What outcome are we trying to change?
- Is a specific narrowing limiting blood flow in a way that explains my symptoms?
- How much symptom improvement is realistic after PCI?
- What are the expected benefits, risks, and reasonable alternatives?
- What happens if we begin with medical therapy and follow-up?

If a scan suggests an important narrowing near the beginning of a major coronary artery, angiography may clarify it. If pressure measurements show that the narrowing does not limit blood flow and the patient has no limiting angina, medical therapy and follow-up may be the better choice.

I do not judge a procedure as good or bad in the abstract. I ask whether it fits the problem in front of us. For my mother, it did. For another patient, it may not. Either way, the decision needs a clear goal, an honest discussion of risk, and room for the uncertainty that remains after the numbers are explained. With or without a procedure, the medicine plan still matters. Chapter 14 explains what each medicine is there to do.

FLOW PRACTICE · NAME THE PROCEDURE'S JOB

Before a planned procedure, ask what outcome it is expected to improve in your case: symptoms, longer-term outcomes, or both. Then ask about the reasonable alternatives.

FLOW TAKEAWAY · CHAPTER 13

Use urgency and goal to interpret a procedure: rescue heart muscle in an acute blockage, relieve symptoms in stable disease, and pair either with system-wide prevention. Before a planned stent or bypass, ask which problem it is meant to solve and what long-term treatment will still be needed afterward.
Use next: Flow Tool 9, Questions Before a Planned Test or Procedure.

CHAPTER 14

Heart Medicines: What Job Does Each One Do?

A patient sets a gallon-size zip-top bag of pill bottles on my desk and asks the question almost everyone eventually asks: "Do I really need all of these?" It is a fair question, and it deserves a real answer rather than a lecture on compliance.

A medication list should be a plan, not an inventory. Some medicines treat what you feel today. Others protect you quietly years from now. Some reduce plaque-related risk across the vascular system. Antiplatelet medicines act on platelets, while anticoagulants act mainly on clotting proteins. Other medicines relieve fluid, support a weakened heart, or control symptoms and rhythm.

The right medicines do more than move numbers on a report. Their value comes from the job they do. Patients also need to know how long that job is expected to last, how benefit and safety will be followed, and what to do when something changes.

Different Medicines, Different Jobs

THE JOB	MEDICINE AND PURPOSE
Lower risk from artery plaque	**Statins and other cholesterol-lowering medicines** Lower LDL cholesterol and ApoB to reduce the risk of heart attack and stroke.
Prevent or treat certain blood clots	**Antiplatelet and anticoagulant medicines** Prescribed for different conditions. They are not interchangeable, and both can increase bleeding risk.
Protect the heart and kidneys	**Heart-failure and blood-pressure medicines** May lower blood pressure, remove excess fluid, or protect the heart and kidneys. Some require blood tests.
Relieve symptoms or manage rhythm	**Beta blockers and other medicines** May ease chest discomfort or palpitations and help control heart rate or rhythm.

MEDICINE SAFETY

Before you start, stop, or combine a heart medicine, ask your clinician or pharmacist.

ASK ABOUT THE JOB

What is this medicine doing for me? How long is that job expected to last? How will we know it is helping safely?

Figure 14.1 · Different Medicines, Different Jobs. A medicine can lower plaque-related risk, prevent or treat certain clots, protect the heart and kidneys, or control symptoms and rhythm. Some medicines do more than one job.

Lower Risk From Artery Plaque

Statins lower the number of cholesterol-carrying particles available to enter the artery wall. LDL cholesterol is the standard measure; ApoB can add useful information in selected patients. Statins reduce heart attacks and strokes, slow plaque growth, and can help make existing plaque less likely to cause trouble.

When I choose the intensity of cholesterol lowering, I start with two questions: How high is this person's untreated risk, and how far does the level need to fall? A prior heart attack, known artery disease, extensive plaque, diabetes, kidney disease, or inherited very high cholesterol usually calls for more intensive lowering than primary prevention in someone at lower risk.

Using Cholesterol-Lowering Medicines in Real Life

For many patients, a tolerated statin is the starting medicine. Muscle symptoms deserve careful assessment rather than dismissal. Serious muscle or liver injury is rare but can occur. Statins can slightly raise blood glucose in susceptible people, while their cardiovascular benefit often remains greater. Large studies have not shown that statins cause dementia.

If symptoms appear, I do not dismiss them. We look for a plan the patient can tolerate.

EVIDENCE SNAPSHOT 14.1

How Statin Therapy Changed Risk

HPS · THE LANCET, 2002; PROVE-IT · NEW ENGLAND JOURNAL OF MEDICINE, 2004

WHAT WAS STUDIED

HPS compared simvastatin with placebo in 20,536 adults at high cardiovascular risk. PROVE-IT compared intensive atorvastatin with moderate pravastatin in 4,162 people soon after an acute coronary syndrome.

WHAT RESEARCHERS FOUND

HPS Major vascular events fell from 25.2% to 19.8% over about five years, or roughly five fewer people in every 100.

PROVE-IT The trial's combined outcome fell from 26.3% to 22.4% over two years, or roughly four fewer people in every 100.

WHAT THIS MEANS

Statins lower cardiovascular events. After an acute event, more intensive LDL lowering can add protection when appropriate and tolerated.

> **IMPORTANT LIMIT**
> The trials enrolled different populations, used different outcomes, and followed patients for different lengths of time. Their percentages should not be compared directly or treated as a personal forecast.

The benefit comes from fewer cardiovascular events, not simply a better laboratory number.

SOURCES Heart Protection Study Collaborative Group, The Lancet, 2002; Cannon et al., New England Journal of Medicine, 2004.

If the risk-based goal is not reached or a statin is not tolerated, options include a different statin or schedule, the pills ezetimibe or bempedoic acid, an injectable PCSK9-blocking medicine, inclisiran, or a combination. Inclisiran lowers LDL cholesterol, but unlike the injectable PCSK9-blocking medicines evolocumab and alirocumab, whether it reduces cardiovascular events remains under study. Report symptoms and adjust the plan with your clinician rather than stopping silently.

Prevent or Treat Certain Blood Clots

After a Heart Attack, Unstable Event, or Stent

After many stent procedures, treatment begins with aspirin plus a second antiplatelet medicine such as clopidogrel, ticagrelor, or prasugrel. The exact combination and duration depend on why the stent was placed, bleeding risk, and the procedure. Some patients later continue one antiplatelet medicine rather than two.

Clots That Can Travel to the Brain or Lungs

Anticoagulants such as apixaban, rivaroxaban, and warfarin act mainly on clotting proteins, while antiplatelet medicines act on platelets. They are used for AFib and for some clots that form in deep leg veins or travel to the lungs. The two categories are not interchangeable. For anyone with a mechanical heart valve, and for people with AFib who have moderate-to-severe narrowing of the mitral valve caused by rheumatic disease, warfarin is generally used rather than a direct oral anticoagulant.

Ask what to do if a dose is late or missed, and do not double a dose unless the instructions specifically say so. Report black stools, vomiting or coughing blood, red or brown urine, or prolonged bleeding.

Seek prompt medical advice after a significant fall or any head injury, even if you initially feel well. Call 911 for severe bleeding, fainting, or signs of stroke.

CRITICAL SAFETY RULE

After a recent stent, do not stop any prescribed antiplatelet medicine without direct guidance from the prescribing cardiology team. Do not start or stop aspirin based on this book. Confirm the intended regimen and duration with your clinician.

Treat High Blood Pressure

Common first-line blood-pressure medicines include thiazide-type diuretics (water pills), long-acting calcium-channel blockers, angiotensin-converting enzyme (ACE) inhibitors, and angiotensin receptor blockers (ARBs). Kidney function, urine albumin, heart failure, angina, rhythm, sodium and potassium levels, pregnancy potential, side effects, and distance from goal all help guide the choice.

ACE inhibitors, ARBs, and a related heart-failure class called angiotensin receptor–neprilysin inhibitors (ARNIs) are not used during pregnancy. The best blood-pressure medicine is the one that fits the rest of the patient's medical picture, not simply the one that lowers a number.

Why a Weakened Heart May Need Several Medicines

Patients often ask, "If all four medicines treat heart failure, why do I need more than one?" Each pathway protects the heart through a different route; one usually cannot stand in for another. You do not need to memorize the names, only why the team is trying to cover more than one pathway.

For many eligible people with reduced pumping strength, these four pathways form the core of treatment. Care teams often begin them over days to weeks, then adjust doses as blood pressure, kidney function, potassium, fluid status, symptoms, and tolerance allow.

Four Foundational Medicine Pathways

ARNI, or an ACE inhibitor or ARB

Relaxes blood vessels and reduces hormone signals that strain a weakened heart. These are alternatives within one pathway, not medicines to combine. The team watches blood pressure, kidney function, potassium, cough, and swelling. A switch from an ACE inhibitor to an ARNI requires a clinician-directed safety gap.

A heart-failure beta blocker

Slows the heart's response to stress hormones, helps it work more efficiently, and lowers the risks of death and hospitalization. The team watches heart rate, blood pressure, dizziness, fatigue, and fluid buildup. The dose usually rises gradually. Do not stop it suddenly.

A mineralocorticoid receptor antagonist (MRA)

Blocks a hormone that promotes salt retention and harmful heart changes. The team watches potassium and kidney function. Do not add a potassium supplement or potassium-containing salt substitute unless the care team approves it.

A sodium-glucose cotransporter 2 (SGLT2) inhibitor

Lowers heart-failure hospitalization and cardiovascular-death risk and can protect kidney function, whether or not the patient has diabetes. The team watches fluid status, kidney function, and signs of genital yeast infection.

Ask when to pause an SGLT2 inhibitor during serious illness, prolonged fasting, or before a procedure.

A Water Pill Has a Different Job

A loop diuretic, often called a water pill, relieves congestion and breathlessness by helping the body remove excess salt and water. It can relieve congestion quickly; the four foundational pathways provide a different kind of long-term protection. The care team may monitor weight, blood pressure, kidney function, electrolytes, and symptoms of too much or too little fluid.

When Pumping Strength Is Mildly Reduced or Preserved

When ejection fraction is above 40 percent, the plan differs from the four-pathway approach used when pumping strength is more clearly reduced. SGLT2 inhibitors can reduce heart-failure events for many eligible people with mildly reduced or preserved pumping strength, while loop diuretics relieve fluid buildup.

Other treatment is matched to the cause, ejection-fraction range, symptoms, and associated conditions such as high blood pressure, atrial fibrillation, kidney disease, diabetes, obesity, coronary disease, or valve disease. Some people, especially those near the lower end of this range, may also benefit from additional heart-failure medicines.

If pumping strength improves after previously being reduced, do not stop heart-failure medicines simply because the ejection fraction is better. Treatment is generally continued to reduce the risk of relapse unless the heart-failure team changes the plan.

Some Medicines Cross Categories

SGLT2 inhibitors can reduce hospitalizations for heart failure and slow kidney disease even when glucose lowering is not their main purpose. Some glucagon-like peptide-1 (GLP-1) receptor agonists reduce cardiovascular events in defined high-risk groups. That is why labels such as "diabetes drug" or "weight-loss drug" can be misleading: the same medicine may protect the heart or kidneys for a separate reason.

Relieve Symptoms or Manage Rhythm

Nitrates must not be combined with medicines for erectile dysfunction, such as sildenafil or tadalafil, because blood pressure can fall dangerously. Chapter 15 discusses this in the context of returning to intimacy.

EVIDENCE IN CONTEXT 14.2

Beta Blockers After a Heart Attack When Pumping Strength Is Normal

Five modern trials included 17,801 people after a heart attack with an ejection fraction of at least 50% and no other reason to take a beta blocker. Over a median of 3.6 years, routine beta-blocker therapy did not reduce the combined outcome of death, another heart attack, or heart failure.

Do not read this as "beta blockers do not work." They remain important when they have another job, including reduced pumping strength or heart failure, angina, selected rhythm disorders, or another indication. Ask why yours was prescribed and whether that reason still applies. Do not stop it abruptly.

SOURCE Kristensen et al., NEJM, 2026.

Before You Stop or Hold a Medicine

Stopping a medicine can have drug-specific consequences. Early interruption of antiplatelet therapy can cause a stent clot. Other abrupt changes may cause rebound symptoms or worsen the condition being treated.

Some medicines do need temporary holds during illness or before a procedure. Follow the plan for that drug, call the prescribing team when unsure, and do not double a missed dose unless instructed. Side effects, cost, pill burden, and a preference for lifestyle treatment all deserve a conversation rather than a silent stop.

By the time the patient with the gallon bag leaves my office, I do not expect them to remember every drug class. I want them to know why each bottle is there and what to do when something changes.

For each medicine, be able to answer five questions:

- What is this medicine for?
- Is it expected to be short-term, long-term, or still being decided?
- How will its benefit and safety be followed?
- Which side effects mean I should call?
- What should I do if I miss a dose or need a procedure?

A procedure or prescription is not the end of treatment. The next part turns to daily life: recovering after an event, making the first ninety days workable, and keeping the plan going for years.

FLOW PRACTICE · KNOW EACH MEDICINE'S JOB

On your medication list, write each medicine's job in a few words. Circle any one you do not understand and ask before changing, skipping, or stopping it.

FLOW TAKEAWAY · CHAPTER 14

A medicine list should read like a plan, not an inventory. Know the purpose, expected duration, monitoring, and stop-or-hold instructions for each medicine. If a medicine is hard to tolerate or afford, ask the prescribing team to adjust the plan before you stop it or begin missing doses.

Use next: Flow Tool 2, My Medication Plan.

PART V

Recovery and the Plan Ahead

Action

Begin with the chapter that matches where you are: recovery after an event, stable prevention, or life beyond ninety days.

CHAPTER 15

Recovery After a Heart Event: Body, Mind, and Daily Life

Procedures and test results can tell you a great deal about what happened to your heart. They cannot capture the uncertainty that follows an event, your first walk around the block, or the moment you wonder whether an ordinary sensation is normal recovery or a warning.

Recovery is medical, physical, and emotional, and each part deserves a plan. A scan can tell you that an artery is open. It cannot tell you how to stop bracing every time you feel your own heartbeat.

Before discharge, or as soon afterward as practical, leave with clear answers:

- Which symptoms require emergency care?
- Whom do I call for non-emergency questions?
- Which medicines must not be interrupted, and what do I do after a missed dose?
- What wound or access-site instructions apply?
- What activity is safe now?
- When are follow-up and cardiac rehabilitation scheduled?

Bring a family member or trusted person when you can. Recovery is easier when the people around you understand the plan and know the difference between useful support and overprotection.

Cardiac Rehab Is Part of Treatment

Cardiac rehabilitation is a structured program of supervised exercise, education, risk-factor management, and support. It is not simply permission to go to a gym. The team evaluates how your heart responds to activity, helps rebuild strength safely, and works with you on medicines, blood pressure, nutrition, tobacco, sleep, and confidence.

A complete program also pays attention to mood, social support, access to care, and the practical barriers that keep people from participating: work, transportation, caregiving, cost, pain, disability, or fear of another event.

People may be referred after a heart attack, coronary stent, bypass surgery, stable angina, or selected heart-failure diagnoses. Eligibility, timing, and insurance coverage vary. Some patients can use home-based, virtual, or hybrid programs with appropriate oversight. If rehabilitation is not offered after an event or procedure, ask whether you qualify and why. The best program is one you can attend safely and consistently.

EVIDENCE SNAPSHOT 15.1

Why Cardiac Rehabilitation Still Matters

CaReMATCH · EUROPEAN JOURNAL OF PREVENTIVE CARDIOLOGY, 2026

WHAT WAS STUDIED

Researchers combined individual results from 4,975 people in eight modern trials of exercise-based cardiac rehabilitation. Nearly all were recovering after a heart attack.

WHAT RESEARCHERS FOUND

People assigned to rehabilitation had fewer hospitalizations for any cause and for heart-related reasons, and reported modestly better quality of life through 12 months. The analysis did not detect a difference in survival.

WHAT THIS MEANS

Recovery does not end when the procedure or hospital stay is over. A structured rehabilitation program can still improve what happens next.

IMPORTANT LIMIT
Only eight of 30 eligible trials supplied individual results. Follow-up was relatively short, and the people enrolled may not represent everyone seen in routine practice.

Cardiac rehabilitation still adds value in the era of modern heart care.
RECOVERY IS PART OF TREATMENT

SOURCE CaReMATCH, European Journal of Preventive Cardiology, 2026.

EVIDENCE IN CONTEXT 15.2

Emotional Recovery

Depression, anxiety, and post-traumatic stress can occur after a heart event. Treatment can improve emotional health and quality of life. It should be offered because the person is suffering and because recovery depends on more than an angiogram—not sold as a cardiovascular cure.

SADHART provided reassuring cardiac-safety evidence for sertraline after a heart attack or unstable angina. It did not show that sertraline prevents another cardiac event, and it does not make sertraline right for everyone.

Medication choice should account for the diagnosis, prior response, bleeding risk, heart rhythm, kidney or liver function, and interactions with heart medicines.

SOURCES Levine et al., Circulation, 2025; Glassman et al., JAMA, 2002.

SAFETY · DO NOT ASSUME IT IS "JUST ANXIETY"
Anxiety can cause chest tightness, breathlessness, sweating, and a racing heart. So can heart problems. A prior anxiety diagnosis does not make new, severe, or worsening symptoms safe to ignore. Follow the emergency plan your team gave you.

If you are thinking about suicide or feel unable to stay safe, get immediate help. In the United States, call or text 988. Call 911 if danger is immediate. Elsewhere, use your local crisis or emergency service.

Stress, Grief, and Takotsubo

The heart and nervous system communicate constantly. Acute grief and severe stress can temporarily raise cardiovascular risk. Rarely, intense physical or emotional stress can trigger Takotsubo syndrome, sometimes called stress cardiomyopathy or broken-heart syndrome.

Takotsubo can cause chest pain, ECG changes, and sudden heart-muscle weakness, mimicking a heart attack. It often improves, but it is not something to diagnose at home. Its symptoms require urgent evaluation because a heart attack and other emergencies must first be ruled out.

Returning to Activity, Work, and Intimacy

Recovery should expand your life, and the timing is individual. Ask for specific guidance about exercise and lifting, driving, returning to work, travel, and sexual activity. Ask separately about procedure-site or surgical restrictions. Make sure you know which symptoms mean "stop" and which mean "call for help."

Driving restrictions may also be governed by local rules after certain events or procedures, so ask specifically rather than assuming. Written guidance is easier to follow than a vague instruction to "take it easy."

Sexual activity is a common concern and an appropriate medical question. For many stable patients, it can resume as recovery progresses; the timing is individual.

Medicines for erectile dysfunction must never be combined with nitrates such as nitroglycerin because the combination can cause a dangerous fall in blood pressure.

If chest symptoms occur during sex, stop and follow your emergency plan, and tell emergency clinicians what medicines you have taken. Recovery can also affect desire, comfort, body image, energy, and relationships. The conversation should not be limited to men or to one type of medicine.

Confidence Returns by Practice

Waiting for every doubt to disappear before becoming active can keep recovery stalled. Cardiac rehabilitation offers a safer place to test the body and rebuild trust in it. Small, repeatable steps often restore confidence better than reassurance alone.

Recovery is rarely smooth. Fatigue, medicine adjustments, poor sleep, or an anniversary of the event can still produce difficult days. One difficult day does not mean your recovery has failed. It may simply be a reason to rest, use the plan, or ask for review.

FLOW TAKEAWAY · CHAPTER 15

Recovery includes what the scan cannot show. Cardiac rehabilitation can help restore function and confidence, and depression, anxiety, or trauma symptoms deserve treatment. Ask directly about exercise, work, driving, travel, intimacy, and the emotional effects of what happened. The goal is a safe return to a full life.

Use next: Flow Tool 3, After a Heart Attack or Stent, and Flow Tool 13, A Quick Guide for Family and Caregivers.

CHAPTER 16

The First 90 Days: Stabilize, Build, Review

The hospital sends you home with a folder, a new list of medicines, and a body you are no longer sure you can trust. The monitors are gone. The nurses are gone. What is left is an ordinary house that suddenly feels like a place where something could go wrong, along with a quiet wish for someone to tell you what to do first.

Not every reader begins here. Some begin with a scan, a blood-pressure pattern, or a laboratory result. The starting points differ, but the need is the same: a clear order for what comes next.

What Can Change in the First 90 Days

The first ninety days are a checkpoint: long enough to learn how the plan works in daily life, rebuild capacity, and fix what is unsafe or unworkable. Plaque and recovery move on a longer clock. New symptoms or a possibly unsafe medicine still require attention before the scheduled review.

Two Different Starting Points

This framework serves two groups of readers, and their medical instructions are not identical.

After an event, procedure, or hospitalization, discharge instructions, wound or access-site care, medicine safety, early follow-up, and cardiac rehabilitation come first.

For stable prevention without a recent event, the first step is to confirm the diagnosis and risk priorities, set a baseline, and decide which changes and measurements are worth following.

In either case, do not try to manage every risk factor with equal urgency on the first day. Start with the decisions that carry the greatest safety or treatment consequence.

Progress will not appear everywhere at once. Blood pressure and laboratory values may change before fitness or confidence does. Symptoms may ease while treatment is still needed to lower long-term risk. A difficult week may reflect poor sleep, illness, grief, pain, or a medicine problem rather than failure of the whole plan.

The first ninety days show what is changing and where the plan needs adjustment.

The Wrong Early Scoreboard

A repeat scan is usually the wrong early scoreboard. Expecting a repeat calcium score or plaque image to prove progress after a few months is like asking for the final score in the second inning. Treatment can be working even when an image has not changed, and some imaging measures are not designed to track short-term response at all.

An off-target blood pressure or laboratory result still matters. Judge each measure by the question it was chosen to answer. At the ninety-day review, ask what the chosen measures show rather than whether plaque has disappeared.

The First 90 Days

Stabilize · Build · Review

Three phases. One adaptable care plan.

1 DAYS 1–30

SAFETY & STABILIZATION

- Know each medicine and the warning signs
- Keep follow-up and rehabilitation appointments
- Stay within your cleared activity level

2 DAYS 31–60

BUILD CAPACITY SAFELY

- Continue rehabilitation or adapted movement
- Review symptoms and medicine tolerance
- Address sleep, food, mood, pain, cost, and access

3 DAYS 61–90

REVIEW & ADJUST

- Gather only the measurements that are due
- Review symptoms, function, benefit, and burden
- Decide what continues, changes, and comes next

THE CLINICAL RULE

Ninety days is a checkpoint, not a biological deadline or proof that plaque is safe.

Figure 16.1 · The 90-Day Plan. The first month emphasizes safety and stabilization, the second builds capacity, and the third reviews progress and adjusts the plan.

At ninety days, do not grade the plan as a success or failure. Review what has become easier, where the plan repeatedly breaks down, and what support or adjustment would make it safer to continue. Direction matters more than perfection, but direction still needs honest review.

Make sure the plan names:

- Medicines and the job of each
- Warning signs and whom to contact
- Home measurements assigned to me
- Laboratory tests due and who reviews them
- Activity restrictions and rehabilitation plan
- Follow-up date
- Barriers we need to solve

A test is not fully followed up until someone knows who will review the result and what happens next.

Make the Plan Easier to Repeat

Good intentions are easier to sustain when they are attached to a simple system: a pill organizer beside the coffee maker, a blood-pressure log on the table, transportation arranged before rehabilitation, or an affordable food plan that fits the household.

Repeating the plan gives you and your care team information that a brief burst of effort cannot provide.

No routine works perfectly. Genes, disease severity, treatment response, and life circumstances still matter. When a routine repeatedly breaks down, ask what got in the way and what would make the next attempt easier. Those barriers belong in the treatment plan.

Days 1–30: Safety and Stabilization

The first month is for making the plan understandable and workable. After an event or procedure, the treating team's instructions come first. The 90-day review is a checkpoint, not the first follow-up; use the timing in your discharge plan. Start with a few priorities: take medicines safely, know which symptoms require urgent care, attend follow-up, and move at a level your team approves.

When a plan is hard to follow, look for the reason. Pain, cost, side effects, low mood, caregiving, transportation, and unclear instructions are medical barriers, not evidence that a patient does not care.

Medication safety comes before optimization. Use a pill organizer, reminder, or another system that fits your life. Know why each medicine is present and who prescribed it. If you miss a dose, follow the label or ask a pharmacist or clinician; do not double the next dose unless told to.

Antiplatelet therapy after a recent stent requires special care and must never be interrupted without direct guidance from the prescribing cardiology team. Ask before adding any over-the-counter pain reliever, cold medicine, herbal product, or supplement, since some can raise bleeding, blood pressure, fluid retention, kidney stress, or cardiovascular risk.

Days 31–60: Build Capacity Safely

The second month is a reasonable time to continue building capacity if recovery is stable and the plan allows. Capacity means being able to do more of ordinary life with less difficulty: walking farther, climbing stairs more comfortably, carrying groceries, returning to work, or recovering more quickly after activity.

Build frequency and duration before chasing intensity. Start from the activity plan your team gave you. The pace depends on recovery, symptoms, fitness, disability, heart function, and the procedure you had. Some movement is usually better than none, and adapted activity counts.

Days 61–90: Review and Adjust

By the final month, the plan should be familiar enough to evaluate. Make notes about symptoms, daily function, rehabilitation, medicine tolerance, cost, sleep, mood, and the barriers that remain. Confirm which measurements are due and who will review them.

Do not wait until Day 90 for new, worsening, or severe symptoms.

Table 16.1 · Measures That Can Guide the 90-Day Review

Measure	What it can show, when to review it, and its limits
Home blood pressure	Shows the pattern outside the clinic and response to treatment. Use a correctly collected series or average when assigned; one reading does not define control.
LDL-C, non-HDL-C (total cholesterol minus HDL-C), or ApoB	Shows response to lipid-lowering treatment. It is commonly checked about 4–12 weeks after treatment starts or changes, then at an interval based on risk and the plan. A lower value does not prove plaque has shrunk.
A1c	Estimates glucose exposure over the prior two to three months when diabetes or prediabetes management calls for it. It does not show day-to-day variation.
Kidney function, sodium, and potassium	Helps assess safety and response for selected medicines and conditions. Timing depends on the drug, dose, kidney function, and clinical situation.
Symptoms and daily function	Shows whether recovery is improving, stable, or losing ground. Review throughout recovery and sooner when symptoms worsen. Feeling better does not remove long-term risk.
Cardiac rehabilitation or activity	Shows participation, exercise response, and functional progress. Review with the rehabilitation or clinical team; exercise minutes alone do not measure the whole recovery.
Imaging	Answers a defined structural or diagnostic question. Repeat it when a new result could change care, not simply to certify that plaque is stable.

Measure	What it can show, when to review it, and its limits
Pulse, rhythm log, or wearable alert	May reveal a recurring pattern that deserves confirmation. A consumer device does not provide a complete diagnosis or capture every rhythm.
Weight and fluid symptoms for selected heart-failure patients	May provide an early warning of fluid buildup when a personal monitoring plan has been assigned. One reading alone does not define fluid status.

Match the Measure to the Question

At the 90-day review, bring the medication list, requested home readings, symptom notes, questions, and any barriers. Leave with four answers:

- What is working and should continue?
- What needs to change or be clarified?
- What needs attention now?
- When is the next review, and what should happen before then?

FLOW TAKEAWAY · CHAPTER 16

The first ninety days are a planning framework: stabilize, build, and review. The phases overlap. Take medicines safely, close the gaps after discharge or diagnosis, rebuild function at an appropriate pace, and measure only what can improve a decision. Leave the review knowing what continues, what changes, what needs attention now, and when the plan will be reviewed again.

Use next: Flow Tool 8, The 90-Day Flow Dashboard.

CHAPTER 17

Flow for the Rest of Your Life: Beyond 90 Days

I see the shift at follow-up. Early on, patients can name every dose and every appointment. Months later, the early urgency has faded, life has filled back in, and the refill that once felt urgent is suddenly three days late.

That is human, not a character flaw. It is also the point at which protection can quietly slip.

Ninety days is long enough to begin building and testing a system. It is not long enough to know whether that system will survive every season of ordinary life. The real test is the years that follow: a bad flu, a funeral, a move, a new grandchild, a layoff, a hospital stay, or a change in mobility. Beyond ninety days, the challenge is no longer starting a plan. It is keeping it workable through real life.

The Long Middle

When I build a long-term plan, I do not want urgency or motivation to be the only fuel. Both have an expiration date. What lasts is protection attached to stable routines: the refill reminder, the regular walk, and the follow-up scheduled before the patient leaves.

If treatment becomes burdensome, costly, or hard to tolerate, we look for an adjustment that preserves its purpose.

When prevention works, nothing dramatic happens. You may see no sign or proof of the crisis that was avoided. That quiet can make treatment feel unnecessary, but it is not a reason to stop.

When Life Interrupts the Plan

FLOW TRUTH

Life will interrupt the routine. The plan should make clear what cannot safely wait, what may need temporary adjustment, and how to restart the rest.

The Never-Miss-Twice Rule

A useful rule for ordinary routines is "never miss twice." Missed a walk today? Return tomorrow if it is safe. Had a poor night of sleep? Protect the next one. Ate outside your usual pattern? Let the next meal be ordinary.

The point is not perfection. It is keeping one disrupted day from becoming a new baseline.

Medication doses are different. Follow the drug-specific missed-dose instructions or ask a pharmacist or clinician, and never double a dose unless instructed.

Illness or poor intake: Some medicines must continue, while others may need a clinician-directed hold. Antiplatelet therapy after a stent must never be stopped without cardiology guidance. Ask for written sick-day instructions for medicines that may need adjustment during dehydration, poor intake, surgery, or acute illness.

Travel: Keep medicines in your carry-on with a current medication list, and pack extra doses in case of delay. Ask before the trip about dosing across time zones when timing matters.

Caregiving or grief: Protect the smallest sustainable routines, accept help, and remember that new cardiac symptoms still deserve care even when your attention is on someone else.

Retirement, a move, or another loss of structure: Much of what protects you may be hidden inside the routine, such as the commute that doubles as a walk, the workday that anchors meals, or the bedtime tied to tomorrow morning. When that scaffolding disappears, rebuild it on purpose: a daily walk, a regular mealtime, or a reason to be somewhere in the morning.

Cost: Do not ration medicine in silence. A generic, a different drug, an assistance program, or another plan may be available, but the conversation needs to happen before doses are missed.

The goal is not to avoid every disruption. It is to notice the drift and return before one hard week becomes abandonment of the whole plan.

What Long-Term Review Should Cover

At long-term visits, I ask whether the plan still fits: what has changed, what remains worth doing, and what has become too hard or unnecessary. The interval depends on the diagnoses, medicines, recent events, and symptoms.

Review:

- Symptoms and daily function
- The reason, dose, duration, tolerance, and cost of each medicine
- Blood pressure, cholesterol, glucose, kidney function, and other assigned measurements
- Tobacco or nicotine use and quit support
- Sleep and sleep apnea
- Activity, strength, falls, and rehabilitation
- Mood and support
- Pending referrals and who is responsible for following them

When things are stable, follow-up may be less frequent. A good follow-up plan names the next checkpoint: what will be measured, who will review it, and which finding should bring you back sooner.

Arrange an earlier review for:

- New or worsening symptoms
- A hospitalization or procedure
- Sustained palpitations, repeated wearable alerts, or another suspected rhythm change
- A major change in kidney function, blood pressure, glucose, weight, or strength
- A new medicine that changes bleeding, kidney, or rhythm risk
- Side effects or cost barriers that are causing you to miss treatment

Contact the team during pregnancy planning or pregnancy, and before beginning or changing menopausal hormone therapy.

Simplifying Treatment Safely

A shorter medicine list can be a worthy goal, but simplification starts with purpose: What protection would be lost if this drug were stopped?

A better laboratory value may be evidence that treatment is working, not that it has become unnecessary. Review any dose reduction or medicine stop with the prescribing clinician and agree on monitoring. If several specialists are involved, keep one current list and identify who will reconcile conflicting instructions.

The goal is not the shortest medicine list. It is the simplest plan you can live with without giving up protection that matters.

FLOW PRACTICE · SCHEDULE THE NEXT CHECKPOINT

Before you leave your next visit, put the recommended follow-up on your calendar or set a reminder to arrange it. Move the review sooner if symptoms, medicines, or health change.

FLOW TAKEAWAY · CHAPTER 17

Beyond ninety days, protection becomes a maintenance practice: keep the plan workable, return after interruptions, and move the next review forward when symptoms, medicines, health, or life change. Your long-term protection is built in the ordinary days between visits.

Use next: Flow Tool 12, Flow Maintenance Checklist Beyond 90 Days.

CONCLUSION

Your Heart, Your Flow, Your Future

Again and again, I have watched fear ease when a patient can finally answer two questions: **What is happening, and what do we do next?**

This book has followed both clocks: the fast clock of an emergency, when minutes matter, and the slower clock of cardiovascular health, when choices and treatments over months and years shape risk, recovery, and quality of life.

My mother is well today. I still remember the night before her procedure, when what I knew as a cardiologist did not lessen what I felt as a son. That experience changed the way I speak with patients and families. Medical evidence matters. So do values, relationships, and the life a treatment is meant to protect.

The next time you face a test result or treatment decision, return to a few questions:

- What problem are we trying to solve?
- What can this test or treatment actually change?
- What are its limits?
- What matters most to me?
- When will we review the plan again?

I want you to hear this as both a cardiologist and a son: fear belongs in the room. Understanding cannot erase it, but it can keep fear from making the decision alone.

You do not need to control every variable. You need a plan you understand, a clear next step, and a time to review it.

Your heart is not a mystery to solve once. It is something to care for over time. You will not remember most of the days that protect it. That is exactly the point.

Protection, done well, is almost invisible: the walk after dinner, the pill beside the coffee, the night you chose sleep, the question you brought to an appointment instead of silence. Each moment is small. Together, they improve the odds and give you a clearer role in your own care.

That is Flow.

The Flow Toolkit

Practical Guides for Visits, Tests, and Treatment Decisions

This is a working reference, not something you need to read front to back. Start with the page that matches the decision in front of you. Return whenever a term feels unfamiliar, a result feels confusing, or a decision needs context.

Which Flow Tool Do I Need?

Find the sentence that sounds most like your situation and go straight to that tool. You do not need to complete the others.

Possible emergency? If symptoms are happening now and may be an emergency, call 911. Do not use a worksheet, wearable, or prior test result to decide that a new severe symptom is safe.

SYMPTOMS & RISK	VISITS, RECOVERY & SUPPORT
I'm unsure whether to call 911, call today, or track a known, stable problem. → Flow Tool 6 · Emergency, Same-Day, or Planned Follow-Up	I'm getting ready for an appointment. → Flow Tool 1 · Preparing for Your Visit
My watch flagged possible atrial fibrillation (AFib). See Flow Tool 14, If Your Watch Flags Possible AFib.	I need to understand or organize my medicines. → Flow Tool 2 · My Medication Plan
My stress test was normal, but I still have questions or symptoms. → Flow Tool 4 · Questions After a Normal Stress Test	I'm deciding about a planned test or procedure. See Flow Tool 9, Questions Before a Planned Test or Procedure.
I need to organize symptoms and pregnancy, menopause, autoimmune, or cancer-treatment history. See Flow Tool 5, Women's and Pregnancy-Related Cardiovascular History Guide.	I'm home after a heart attack or stent. → Flow Tool 3 · After a Heart Attack or Stent
I need a seven-day record of symptoms and trends. → Flow Tool 11 · Symptom and Trend Tracker	I'm building or reviewing a 90-day prevention or recovery plan. → Flow Tool 8 · The 90-Day Flow Dashboard
I want to map cardiovascular problems in my family. → Flow Tool 7 · Family Flow Map	I'm beyond 90 days and need a long-term check-in. → Flow Tool 12 · Flow Maintenance Checklist Beyond 90 Days

SYMPTOMS & RISK	VISITS, RECOVERY & SUPPORT
I want to see which cardiovascular risks I may be able to change. See Flow Tool 10, My Cardiovascular Risk Snapshot.	I'm helping someone protect their heart. → Flow Tool 13 · A Quick Guide for Family and Caregivers

Looking for a quick reference? Use the FLOWS Symptom-Description Aid, Quick Test Reference, Medication Summary, or eating and activity guides in this toolkit.

Start Here: Your First Three Moves

When you close this book, do not try to solve everything at once. Begin with these three moves. Seek care promptly for new or worsening symptoms rather than working through a checklist.

Learn Your Blood-Pressure Pattern

If home monitoring is part of your plan, use a validated automatic upper-arm device with the correct cuff size. For 30 minutes before measuring, avoid smoking, caffeine, alcohol, and exercise, and empty your bladder. Sit quietly for at least five minutes with your back supported, feet flat and uncrossed, arm at heart level, cuff on bare skin, and do not talk. Unless your care team says otherwise, take two readings one minute apart, morning and evening, for three to seven days. Record all results and share them with your care team. Do not change medicine because of one isolated reading unless your clinician has given you a specific plan.

Know the Numbers That Shape Your Plan

Know your LDL-C and whether your glucose screening is current. Current guidance recommends measuring Lp(a) at least once in adulthood. Ask whether ApoB would add useful information in your situation; it can be especially helpful when triglycerides are high, diabetes is present, or LDL-C may understate the number of plaque-forming particles. Ask which result matters most for you, what the goal is, and when it should be reviewed.

Ask the Next-Step Question

At your next visit, ask: "What is most likely driving my risk or symptoms, and what should we do next?" Ask what the next test, medicine, or procedure is meant to change, who will review the result, and when. If the plan will not work in your life, explain why; cost, side effects, work, caregiving, mood, pain, or disability may require the plan to change.

Section I: When Clarity and Timing Matter Most

Emergency Shortcut

Call 911 now for any of the following

- Chest pressure, heaviness, squeezing, or tightness that is new and happening now, is severe or worsening, lasts more than a few minutes or repeatedly returns, or occurs at rest or with minimal exertion.
- Chest discomfort accompanied by breathlessness, sweating, nausea, fainting, marked weakness, or discomfort spreading to the arm, jaw, neck, back, or shoulder.
- Sudden severe breathlessness, fainting, or possible stroke signs, including facial drooping, one-sided weakness, or trouble speaking.
- A very fast or irregular heartbeat with dizziness or fainting.

Do not drive yourself, wait to see whether it passes, or assume it is anxiety, reflux, or muscle pain.

Flow Tool 6 is the complete printable guide. It separates emergencies from same-day calls and findings that can be tracked only after they have already been evaluated and a follow-up plan is in place.

Section II: Making Sense of Tests, Symptoms, and Results

Quick Test Reference

What each test answers and what it cannot show.

Test	What question it answers	What it cannot show
ECG (also called EKG)	Your heart's rhythm and electrical activity, including changes that may suggest a current or prior heart injury.	A reassuring ECG does not exclude a heart attack, plaque, or a problem in the heart's smallest vessels.
Calcium score (CAC)	The amount of calcified coronary plaque at the time of the scan, used to refine estimated long-term risk.	Blood flow, noncalcified plaque, or whether plaque is stable.
Stress test	Whether exercise or medicine-induced stress produces signs that part of the heart is not receiving enough blood, plus exercise capacity when measured.	It does not show all plaque, predict which plaque may break open, or rule out every problem in the heart's smallest vessels.

Test	What question it answers	What it cannot show
CT angiogram (CCTA)	Where coronary plaque is, how much is present, whether it is calcified or noncalcified, and the degree of any narrowing.	Whether an individual plaque will rupture or how blood flow changes during ordinary activity. In selected patients, a separate computer analysis of the CT scan may estimate whether a narrowing restricts blood flow.
Invasive angiogram	The pattern of your coronary arteries and the degree of any narrowing.	The angiogram alone does not show what is happening inside plaque or how the smallest vessels function.
Pressure tests called FFR and iFR	An estimate of whether a specific narrowing is likely to limit coronary blood flow.	Risk elsewhere in the arteries, plaque stability, or every small-vessel problem.
Echocardiogram	How well your heart muscle pumps and fills, and how your valves work.	Coronary plaque and arterial biology.

Test	What question it answers	What it cannot show
Selected laboratory tests	Which measurable risk factors or safety issues are present. Depending on the question, this may include LDL-C, non-HDL-C, ApoB, Lp(a), triglycerides, blood sugar or A1c, kidney function, blood salts such as sodium and potassium, and selected inflammation markers.	Exactly where plaque is, whether a specific plaque will rupture, or how coronary blood flow behaves during daily activity.

A normal result means the test was normal for what it measured, not that everything is normal.

The FLOWS Symptom-Description Aid

The FLOWS Symptom-Description Aid helps organize what happened before a visit. It is a communication aid, not a diagnostic test.

- F: Feeling. What did it feel like: pressure, squeezing, heaviness, burning, breathlessness, racing or skipped beats, or unusual fatigue?
- L: Location. Where did you feel it: chest, jaw, neck, back, shoulder, arm, or upper abdomen?
- O: Onset and duration. When did it begin? Was the onset sudden or gradual? How long did it last, and is the pattern changing?
- W: What brings it on or relieves it. Exertion, stress, cold, meals, position, breathing, rest, or prescribed medicine?

- S: Safety signals. Call 911 for new, severe, or worsening chest discomfort; severe breathlessness at rest; fainting; or possible stroke signs such as facial drooping, one-sided weakness, or trouble speaking. Contact your clinician today for other new or worsening patterns.

Symptoms from the heart and from noncardiac causes can overlap. Use FLOWS to describe the pattern clearly, not to decide the cause yourself.

Common Measures and Risk-Based Reference Points

These are common reference points, not a personal prescription. A laboratory's population range is not the same as a treatment goal. Ask which risk category and guideline your care team is using.

Measure	What it tells you	Common reference point	What to ask
LDL-C	The cholesterol carried in LDL particles, which are causally involved in atherosclerosis	Current U.S. guidance uses risk-based goals. Examples include below 100 mg/dL for some borderline- or intermediate-risk primary-prevention patients, below 70 mg/dL for high-risk patients, and below 55 mg/dL for very-high-risk secondary prevention. The category matters.	"What is my risk category, what is my LDL-C goal, and how much reduction are we trying to achieve?"
ApoB	The number of cholesterol-carrying particles that can enter the artery wall and help form plaque	Especially useful when LDL-C may understate the number of plaque-forming particles, including with high triglycerides, diabetes, obesity, or metabolic disease. A single universal ApoB goal does not apply to everyone.	"Would ApoB change my treatment goal or show risk that LDL-C is missing?"

Measure	What it tells you	Common reference point	What to ask
Non-HDL-C	Cholesterol carried in all potentially plaque-forming particles	Often used when ApoB is not available. A common reference is about 30 mg/dL above the LDL-C goal, but the treatment plan remains risk-based.	"Is non-HDL-C a useful treatment measure for me?"
Blood pressure	The pressure load on the heart, arteries, kidneys, and brain	Below 130/80 mm Hg is a common goal for many adults. Goals may need adjustment for dizziness or a blood-pressure drop when standing, falls, physical frailty, pregnancy, or other clinical circumstances.	"What home average should I aim for, and which readings should I report?"

Measure	What it tells you	Common reference point	What to ask
A1c	A blood test estimating average blood sugar over two to three months	Below 7% is a common goal for many nonpregnant adults with diabetes, but the goal may be lower or higher depending on age, medicines, risk of dangerously low blood sugar, kidney disease, and other conditions.	"What A1c goal gives me the best balance of benefit and safety?"
Lp(a)	A mostly inherited cholesterol-related particle that can raise the risk of plaque-related artery disease and calcium-related narrowing of the aortic valve	Measure at least once in adulthood. A level of 125 nmol/L or higher, or 50 mg/dL or higher, is generally considered a finding that raises risk. The two units are not directly interchangeable.	"Does this result change how intensively we manage LDL-C and my other risks?"

Measure	What it tells you	Common reference point	What to ask
Triglycerides	A measure related to leftover cholesterol-rich particles and metabolic health	Below 150 mg/dL is a common fasting reference point. Treatment depends on the degree of elevation, the risk of inflammation of the pancreas (pancreatitis), diabetes, alcohol, medicines, thyroid status, and cardiovascular risk.	"Do we need to look for a cause, change treatment, or repeat this test while I am fasting?"
hs-CRP	A general marker of inflammation somewhere in the body; it does not identify the source	A persistent value of 2 mg/L or higher can raise estimated risk when measured in a stable state. Infection, injury, autoimmune disease, and other inflammation can raise it.	"Was this measured when I was well, and would the result change a decision?"

Measure	What it tells you	Common reference point	What to ask
CAC score	The burden of calcified coronary plaque at the time of the scan	Interpret the score with age, percentile, symptoms, and overall risk. A score of zero can lower near-term risk in an appropriate asymptomatic adult but does not rule out noncalcified plaque or evaluate symptoms.	"How does this result change prevention, and would repeating it ever change care?"
Kidney measures	Estimated glomerular filtration rate (eGFR) estimates how well the kidneys filter blood; a urine albumin-to-creatinine ratio looks for leakage of the protein albumin into the urine	These are not heart tests, but kidney disease changes cardiovascular risk and medication choices. An abnormal result often needs confirmation and clinical context.	"Does kidney function change my cardiovascular risk, medicine dose, or monitoring plan?"

Reference-Point Note

Do not combine targets from several guidelines into a single hybrid goal. Your clinician should identify the risk category, choose the goal that applies, and tell you when it will be reviewed.

Section III: Treatments, Tools, and Long-Term Strategy

Medication Summary

Antiplatelet medicines: Aspirin and a second antiplatelet medicine, such as clopidogrel or ticagrelor, reduce platelet-related clotting in selected conditions, including after many heart attacks, some episodes of unstable angina, and stent procedures.

Lipid-lowering medicines: Statins lower LDL-C and ApoB and reduce cardiovascular events. Ezetimibe, bempedoic acid, and PCSK9-directed therapies can provide additional lowering for selected patients. The choice depends on diagnosis, baseline risk, response, tolerance, cost, access, and the treatment goal.

Blood-pressure and vascular medicines: ACE inhibitors and ARBs treat high blood pressure and heart failure and protect the kidneys in selected patients. Calcium-channel blockers and nitrates may treat angina or coronary spasm. The choice depends on the diagnosis and required monitoring.

Diuretics: Reduce excess fluid or blood pressure when indicated; monitoring needs vary by drug.

Heart, Kidney and Metabolic Therapies: Sodium-glucose cotransporter 2 (SGLT2) inhibitors improve heart or kidney outcomes for specific indications. Glucagon-like peptide-1 (GLP-1) medicines and dual-incretin medicines are used for selected diabetes or chronic weight-management indications; cardiovascular evidence differs by medicine.

Anticoagulants: Direct oral anticoagulants such as apixaban and rivaroxaban are used for atrial fibrillation and clots in a deep vein or the lungs (venous thromboembolism) in appropriate patients. Warfarin is used for some of those conditions and is the standard anticoagulant for mechanical heart valves. These medicines are not interchangeable with antiplatelets or with one another.

Do not stop or change a prescribed heart medicine on your own. Contact the prescribing team or pharmacist, and seek urgent help for a suspected serious reaction.

Before You Add an Over-the-Counter Product

Ask a clinician or pharmacist before adding an over-the-counter pain reliever, cold medicine, herbal product, or supplement.

Nonsteroidal anti-inflammatory drugs (NSAIDs), such as ibuprofen, can increase the risk of heart attack, heart failure, stroke, gastrointestinal bleeding, higher blood pressure or fluid retention, and kidney injury. Risk can be greater with higher doses, longer use, or anticoagulant or antiplatelet therapy. Some decongestants can raise blood pressure or heart rate, and supplements can interact with prescription medicines. Ask a clinician or pharmacist before use.

The safest option depends on your diagnoses and current medicines. Bring the actual package or a clear photograph of the label when you ask.

A Clear Look at Supplements

A supplement bottle cannot tell you whether the product works, whether its dose is reliable, or whether it will interact with your medicines. Natural does not mean proven or harmless.

Product	What patients should know
Fish oil and prescription icosapent ethyl	Store-bought omega-3 mixtures and prescription icosapent ethyl are not the same treatment. Store-bought mixtures have not consistently prevented heart attacks or strokes. Prescription icosapent ethyl helped a selected group of high-risk patients with elevated triglycerides. Higher-dose omega-3 products may increase AFib risk in some people.
Red yeast rice	Some products contain a substance chemically identical to lovastatin, but strength and purity vary. They can cause statin-like muscle, liver, kidney, and drug-interaction problems. Do not use red yeast rice as a do-it-yourself statin.
Coenzyme Q10 (CoQ10)	It is often tried for statin-associated muscle symptoms, but trial results are inconsistent. It can interact with medicines, including warfarin. Muscle symptoms deserve a review of timing, other causes, dose, and treatment alternatives.
Niacin	High-dose niacin is no longer a routine add-on to statin treatment. Major trials did not show added cardiovascular benefit and found more side effects. It now has limited specialist-directed roles.
Vitamins, minerals, and antioxidant pills	Treat a confirmed deficiency when appropriate, but routine vitamin D, magnesium, folic acid, B-vitamin, vitamin E, vitamin C, or beta-carotene pills have not broadly prevented cardiovascular events in people without a specific indication.

Supplements do not replace indicated treatment of cholesterol, blood pressure, diabetes, tobacco exposure, or another cardiovascular risk.

Your Habits: From Start to Stability

Use the prompts below as examples, not prescriptions.

Area	Plan	Review
Movement	Follow the activity or rehabilitation plan appropriate to your condition.	Review symptoms, function, and whether progression is safe.
Nutrition	Choose a sustainable pattern that fits your health, culture, and access.	Use clinician- or dietitian-set sodium, fluid, potassium, protein, or carbohydrate goals when needed.
Sleep	Allow a regular sleep opportunity when circumstances permit.	Seek assessment for persistent insomnia, snoring, witnessed pauses, or marked sleepiness.
Stress and coping	Choose one coping practice that is realistic and helpful.	Review what helps; seek care when symptoms are persistent or severe.
Weight and monitoring	Track weight or waist only when it is clinically useful.	Use daily weights when a heart-failure team recommends them.

Individual goals differ. Review what is safe, useful, and sustainable with your care team.

What Should I Eat? A Practical Flow Guide

A Mediterranean-style or similarly plant-forward eating pattern can reduce cardiovascular risk. Favor vegetables, fruit, legumes, whole grains, nuts, unsaturated oils, and appropriate protein sources, with fewer highly processed foods and sugar-sweetened drinks.

The food environment matters. Ultraprocessed products are often inexpensive, convenient, and heavily marketed. Higher intake is associated with more cardiovascular disease, although much of the long-term evidence is observational and the category itself is imperfect. The category describes processing and does not by itself determine the nutritional value of every product: frozen vegetables, canned beans, plain yogurt, and whole-grain bread can be useful. Focus first on repeated choices most likely to matter, such as sugar-sweetened drinks, processed meats, packaged sweets, and salty refined snacks. Replace one frequent item at a time with something you can afford and repeat.

One simple visual guide is the 50/25/25 plate: half vegetables, one-quarter protein, and one-quarter high-fiber carbohydrate. No weighing or measuring is required. It is a flexible starting point, not a prescription; individual needs may change the proportions.

Replace saturated fats with unsaturated fats when possible and avoid industrial trans fats. Fish, poultry, eggs, dairy, and plant proteins can fit in different amounts according to preference, culture, allergies, kidney function, and nutritional needs.

Sodium, fluid, potassium, protein, and carbohydrate targets should reflect blood pressure, heart failure, kidney disease, diabetes, medicines, and access to food. Cooking at home can help some people, but it is not the only way to build a healthy pattern.

There is no cardiovascular reason to start drinking alcohol. If you drink, less is generally better, and some conditions or medicines call for none.

A Sample Day

Use this as an example of the principles on an ordinary plate. Swap freely; the overall pattern matters more than the specific foods.

- Breakfast: Plain Greek yogurt with oats, berries, and walnuts, or eggs with fruit and a high-fiber grain. Protein and fiber can improve fullness and make the meal easier to sustain through the morning.
- Lunch: A big salad or grain bowl built on the 50/25/25 plate: half vegetables and greens, a quarter protein (beans, fish, chicken), a quarter high-fiber carbohydrate (quinoa, farro, sweet potato), dressed with extra-virgin olive oil.
- Snack: Fruit and nuts, hummus and vegetables, or a piece of fruit with cheese. The goal is to arrive at dinner without being ravenous.
- Dinner: About twice a week, choose lower-mercury fish when relevant. On other days, use beans, lentils, poultry, or another protein that fits your needs. Add vegetables and a high-fiber grain or other minimally processed carbohydrate.
- Drinks: Water, coffee, or tea when appropriate.

This sample day is not a rigid diet or calorie prescription. It shows a practical pattern: mostly minimally processed foods, adequate protein, healthy fats, and meal timing you can sustain.

Section IV: Using Flow in Real Life

How to Use Flow With Your Doctor

The best appointments start with a clear question.

Questions that work well include:

- "What problem are we solving today?"
- "Is this about symptoms now, or risk over time?"
- "What does this test tell us, and what can't it tell us?"
- "What are the benefits and risks of acting now versus trying medicine first or scheduling follow-up?"
- "What symptom or result would change the plan?"

Return to the Flow questions when the pieces do not seem to fit: a reassuring test but continuing symptoms, an abnormal scan but no immediate procedure, or several reasonable choices with no obvious winner.

Outside an emergency, some decisions can be made with medicines, follow-up, or planned testing rather than an immediate procedure. Bring what has changed, the question you most need answered, and the tradeoffs that matter to you.

Use the framework to ask better questions, not to diagnose yourself or assume that one result automatically calls for a particular test.

The Flow Tools

WORKSHEETS FOR VISITS, DECISIONS, AND FOLLOW-THROUGH

Use the tool that matches the question in front of you. Fill it in, bring it to the visit, and update it when the plan changes.

PLAN	**Tools 1-3** Visits, medications, and recovery after an event
UNDERSTAND	**Tools 4-6** Unexplained symptoms, women's history, and urgency
BUILD	**Tools 7-10** Family risk, the first 90 days, decisions, and priorities
MAINTAIN	**Tools 11-14** Tracking, long-term review, support, and watch alerts

TOOL 6 IS KEPT NEAR THE FRONT

The emergency and same-day guide appears early in the toolkit so it is easy to find. Later tools should never delay urgent care.

PRINTABLE FLOW TOOL

Flow Tool 1: Preparing for Your Visit

PRINTABLE VERSION

Optional. Bring this with you if it helps.

Bring if available: your current medication list, home readings, recent test reports, and the name of the clinician or person who referred you.

Why I'm Here Today

What changed? What prompted this visit?

____

____

Symptoms or Changes I've Noticed

New symptoms, worsening symptoms, or changes in tolerance:

- ☐ Chest pressure, pain, or discomfort
- ☐ Shortness of breath
- ☐ Fatigue or weakness
- ☐ Lightheadedness or dizziness
- ☐ Palpitations
- ☐ Leg swelling or pain
- ☐ Less able to walk or exercise than usual
- ☐ Something else: ______________________________

flowheartandvascular.com/flow-tools

PRINTABLE FLOW TOOL

Flow Tool 1: Preparing for Your Visit

What I'm Most Concerned About

Naming the concern can help make the decision clearer.

____

____

____

Questions I Want Answered

The one question I most need answered:

____

____

____

- [ ] What might explain my symptoms, and which causes need to be ruled out?
- [ ] Which test, if any, would answer the question?
- [ ] What does this mean for my short-term and long-term risk?
- [ ] What should I do before the next review?
- [ ] What would not help right now?

Next Steps We Agreed On

Tests, if any: ______________________________

Medication changes, if any: ______________________________

Follow-up timing: ______________________________

Bring this sheet to your appointment.

PRINTABLE FLOW TOOL

Flow Tool 2: My Medication Plan

PRINTABLE VERSION

Complete this using your medication list or with your pharmacist. Use one section per medicine. Record missed-dose, sick-day, or procedure instructions only when a clinician or pharmacist has given them to you. Include prescribed medicines, over-the-counter products, vitamins, and supplements. Photocopy these pages if you need more space.

Medicine 1

Medicine, dose, and time: ______________________________

Why I take it: ______________________________

Prescriber: ______________________________

Expected duration or next review, if known: ______________

Missed-dose, sick-day, or procedure instructions I was given:

____

Questions, side effects, cost, or refill concerns:

____

flowheartandvascular.com/flow-tools

PRINTABLE FLOW TOOL

Flow Tool 2: My Medication Plan

Medicine 2

Medicine, dose, and time: ______________________

Why I take it: ______________________

Prescriber: ______________________

Expected duration or next review, if known: ____________

Missed-dose, sick-day, or procedure instructions I was given:

____

Questions, side effects, cost, or refill concerns:

____

Medicine 3

Medicine, dose, and time: ______________________

Why I take it: ______________________

Prescriber: ______________________

Expected duration or next review, if known: ____________

Missed-dose, sick-day, or procedure instructions I was given:

____

Questions, side effects, cost, or refill concerns:

____

____

PRINTABLE FLOW TOOL

Flow Tool 2: My Medication Plan

Medicine 4

Medicine, dose, and time: ______________________

Why I take it: ______________________

Prescriber: ______________________

Expected duration or next review, if known: ____________

Missed-dose, sick-day, or procedure instructions I was given:

____

Questions, side effects, cost, or refill concerns:

____

Medicine 5

Medicine, dose, and time: ______________________

Why I take it: ______________________

Prescriber: ______________________

Expected duration or next review, if known: ____________

Missed-dose, sick-day, or procedure instructions I was given:

____

Questions, side effects, cost, or refill concerns:

____

____

PRINTABLE FLOW TOOL

Flow Tool 2: My Medication Plan

Medicine 6

Medicine, dose, and time: ______

Why I take it: ______

Prescriber: ______

Expected duration or next review, if known: ______

Missed-dose, sick-day, or procedure instructions I was given:

______

Questions, side effects, cost, or refill concerns:

______

PRINTABLE FLOW TOOL

Flow Tool 2: My Medication Plan

Medication Safety

After a stent

Personalized stent-related medication safety advice:

____

____

Anticoagulant safety

Important considerations:

- Take exactly as directed and do not skip doses unless a clinician tells you to.
- Call for guidance before surgery, dental work, or if bleeding, bruising, or falls become a concern.

Warning signs:

- ______________________________________
- ______________________________________

Beta blocker or rhythm-medicine safety

Notes and safety tips:

____

____

PRINTABLE FLOW TOOL

Flow Tool 2: My Medication Plan

Medication Safety

SGLT2 and other diabetes/heart-failure medicine instructions

Instructions and specific guidelines:

____

Potential side effects to monitor: ______________________________

____

Supplement safety

Supplement-related safety considerations:

- [ ] ______________________________
- [ ] ______________________________
- [ ] ______________________________

My Specific Hold / Restart Instructions

Use this area for your care team to enter patient-specific instructions about holding, stopping, or restarting medicines around procedures or illness.

____

____

____

____

PRINTABLE FLOW TOOL

Flow Tool 3: After a Heart Attack or Stent

PRINTABLE VERSION

A heart attack is an injury. A stent treats one site. Recovery and prevention protect the whole cardiovascular system.

SAFETY

Call 911 for severe or uncontrolled bleeding, fainting, new chest pressure, severe breathlessness, or stroke symptoms. Follow your discharge instructions for procedure-site concerns.

Medicines

- Take antiplatelet medicine exactly as prescribed. Do not stop it without direct guidance from the prescribing cardiology team.
- Continue the prescribed statin or other lipid-lowering medicine even when the numbers improve. Ask what low-density lipoprotein cholesterol (LDL-C) goal applies to you.
- Know what to do after a missed dose. Do not double a dose unless instructed.
- Ask before using an anti-inflammatory pain reliever, decongestant, supplement, or herbal product.

flowheartandvascular.com/flow-tools

PRINTABLE FLOW TOOL

Flow Tool 3: After a Heart Attack or Stent

Follow-Up

- My cardiology follow-up date: ____________________
- My primary-care follow-up date: ____________________
- Cardiac rehabilitation referral placed: Yes / No / Not sure
- Whom to call during office hours: ____________________
- Whom to call after hours: ____________________
- Tests, laboratory work, or referrals still pending: ________

Procedure Site or Incision

Follow your discharge instructions. Call 911 if a catheter puncture site swells rapidly or bleeding does not slow with firm pressure. Call your care team for numbness or tingling, a cold or blue limb, increasing bruising or swelling, drainage, fever, increasing pain, or another wound concern. Record any instructions specific to you:

____

____

PRINTABLE FLOW TOOL

Flow Tool 3: After a Heart Attack or Stent

Activity and Recovery

- Activity or lifting restrictions: ____________________
- Driving or work restrictions: ____________________
- Cardiac-rehabilitation start date: ____________________
- Mood, sleep, pain, or support concern to discuss: ______

Rescue Plan

Was nitroglycerin or another rescue medicine prescribed? Yes / No

Instructions I was given:

____

____

Never combine nitroglycerin or another nitrate with sildenafil, tadalafil, vardenafil, avanafil, or riociguat. The combination can cause a dangerous drop in blood pressure. If chest discomfort occurs after taking one of these medicines, call 911. Do not drive. Tell responders what you took and when, and do not take nitroglycerin unless emergency personnel specifically direct you.

PRINTABLE FLOW TOOL

Flow Tool 4: Questions After a Normal Stress Test

PRINTABLE VERSION

A normal result is good news. These questions help you understand what the test settled and how far its reassurance extends.

- What exactly did this test rule out?
- Does it tell us whether I have plaque?
- Can this test predict which plaque will break open or when? (No.)
- If my symptoms continue, what possible cause have we not yet evaluated?
- Should my prevention change based on my overall risk?
- What noncardiac causes should we consider if the heart evaluation does not explain the symptoms?

Remember: A normal stress test means the test did not find evidence that part of the heart was receiving too little blood under the conditions tested. It does not show all plaque that is present without a major blockage or rule out every problem involving the heart's smallest vessels. New or worsening symptoms still require reassessment.

flowheartandvascular.com/flow-tools

PRINTABLE FLOW TOOL

Flow Tool 5: Women's and Pregnancy-Related Cardiovascular History Guide

PRINTABLE VERSION

Symptoms can come from a major coronary blockage, problems in the heart's smallest vessels, coronary spasm, rhythm problems, structural heart disease, or causes outside the heart. Use this page to describe the pattern and identify history that may change risk assessment. It does not diagnose the cause. Pregnancy and ovarian history can be clinically relevant regardless of gender identity.

Describe the Pattern

- [ ] Chest pressure, tightness, heaviness, burning, or discomfort
- [ ] Breathlessness out of proportion to the activity
- [ ] Jaw, neck, back, shoulder, arm, or upper-abdominal discomfort
- [ ] New or unusual fatigue, nausea, sweating, or reduced exercise capacity
- [ ] Symptoms with exertion, emotional stress, cold exposure, or meals
- [ ] Symptoms at rest, overnight, or in the early morning
- [ ] Palpitations, faintness, or near-fainting
- [ ] A new, worsening, or more frequent pattern

flowheartandvascular.com/flow-tools

PRINTABLE FLOW TOOL

Flow Tool 5: Women's and Pregnancy-Related Cardiovascular History Guide

Do not assume a new symptom or palpitation is caused by menopause, anxiety, reflux, or a muscle problem without appropriate evaluation.

History That May Change the Conversation

- ☐ Preeclampsia, gestational hypertension, gestational diabetes, preterm delivery, or another serious pregnancy complication
- ☐ Menopause before age 40 or removal of both ovaries at a young age
- ☐ Polycystic ovary syndrome (PCOS), especially with diabetes, high blood pressure, abnormal cholesterol, or excess weight
- ☐ Autoimmune or chronic inflammatory disease
- ☐ Breast or chest radiation, anthracycline treatment, HER2-directed therapy (used for some breast cancers), or another cancer treatment that can affect the heart or blood vessels
- ☐ Prior spontaneous coronary artery dissection (SCAD, a tear within a coronary artery wall), myocardial infarction with nonobstructive coronary arteries (MINOCA, a heart attack without a major artery blockage), Takotsubo or stress cardiomyopathy, or heart failure related to pregnancy (peripartum cardiomyopathy)

PRINTABLE FLOW TOOL

Flow Tool 5: Women's and Pregnancy-Related Cardiovascular History Guide

History That May Change the Conversation

- [ ] Migraine with aura, meaning temporary visual, sensory, or speech symptoms before or during a migraine, especially when discussing stroke risk or estrogen-containing contraception
- [ ] A strong family history or known high lipoprotein(a), or Lp(a)

Questions to Ask

- Could a major coronary blockage still explain this pattern?
- Could reduced heart-muscle blood flow without a major artery blockage, called ischemia with no obstructive coronary arteries (INOCA), explain this? Possibilities include problems in the smallest coronary vessels, coronary spasm, or more than one mechanism.
- Does my pregnancy, menopause, autoimmune, or cancer-treatment history change prevention or testing?
- If the first test was reassuring but symptoms continue, what question remains unanswered?

Emergency Reminder

For emergency warning signs and timing, use Flow Tool 6.

PRINTABLE FLOW TOOL

Flow Tool 6: Emergency, Same-Day, or Planned Follow-Up

PRINTABLE VERSION

Practical triage, not a substitute for medical advice.

This page helps you sort urgency. It does not replace clinical judgment, and the examples are not exhaustive. If you are unsure whether symptoms could be an emergency, call 911. If the question is nonurgent, call your clinician.

flowheartandvascular.com/flow-tools

PRINTABLE FLOW TOOL

Flow Tool 6: Emergency, Same-Day, or Planned Follow-Up

Call 911 Now

Do not drive yourself. Do not wait to see whether it passes. Do not assume it is anxiety, reflux, or muscle pain.

- Chest pressure, heaviness, squeezing, or tightness that is new and happening now; is severe or worsening; lasts more than a few minutes; or repeatedly returns
- Sudden severe chest or upper-back pain, especially with faintness, sweating, weakness, or a sense that something is seriously wrong
- New chest discomfort or breathlessness happening now at rest or with minimal exertion, especially with sweating, nausea, fainting, or marked weakness
- New pain or pressure spreading to the arm, jaw, neck, back, or shoulder, especially with chest discomfort or breathlessness
- Sudden severe shortness of breath; fainting or near-fainting; or a very fast or irregular heartbeat with dizziness or fainting
- Possible stroke: sudden face droop or numbness or weakness on one side; sudden confusion or trouble speaking or understanding; sudden trouble seeing; sudden trouble walking, dizziness, or loss of balance or coordination; or a sudden severe headache with no known cause. Call 911 immediately.

PRINTABLE FLOW TOOL

Flow Tool 6: Emergency, Same-Day, or Planned Follow-Up

Call Your Clinician the Same Day

Use this tier only if the symptom has completely stopped and no emergency feature above is present. Call your clinician now for same-day guidance. If you cannot reach a clinician promptly, or if the symptom returns, worsens, occurs at rest or with minimal activity, lasts more than a few minutes, or develops any emergency feature, call 911.

Examples: a new exertional pattern of chest pressure or breathlessness that has completely stopped; worsening exercise tolerance; recurrent palpitations without fainting; new or increasing swelling or rapid weight gain; or a concerning medication side effect without emergency signs. Trouble breathing or facial swelling is an emergency.

Blood pressure: Follow your clinician's personal report range. If a home reading is above 180 systolic and/or 120 diastolic, wait at least one minute and repeat it. If it remains this high with chest pain, shortness of breath, back pain, numbness, weakness, vision change, trouble speaking, or another new severe symptom, call 911. Without those symptoms, contact your health care professional promptly. Do not take an extra dose unless instructed. During pregnancy or postpartum, follow the obstetric plan instead: 160 systolic or 110 diastolic is severe and requires immediate contact with the obstetric team or urgent evaluation.

PRINTABLE FLOW TOOL

Flow Tool 6: Emergency, Same-Day, or Planned Follow-Up

Track Until Your Next Visit

Use this tier only when the finding has already been evaluated and you have a plan. Record the pattern and follow your clinician's instructions about when to call or seek urgent care.

- A familiar, unchanged symptom your clinician has already evaluated
- A borderline laboratory result with a planned review
- Stable imaging findings with an agreed follow-up plan
- Difficulty following activity, nutrition, or monitoring plans when the issue is stable and a follow-up plan is already in place

REMINDER

If you are running out of a critical medicine or expect missed doses, especially after a recent stent or while taking an anticoagulant, contact the prescribing team promptly rather than waiting for the next visit.

PRINTABLE FLOW TOOL

Flow Tool 7: Family Flow Map

PRINTABLE VERSION

Record early heart attacks, strokes, rhythm problems, heart-muscle or aortic disease, and sudden death.

YOU, SIBLINGS, AND CHILDREN

	CONDITION	AGE AT ONSET	NOTES
Self			
Sibling(s)			
Child(ren)			

PARENT GENERATION

	CONDITION	AGE AT ONSET	NOTES
Father			
Mother			
Uncle or aunt			
Other relative			

flowheartandvascular.com/flow-tools

PRINTABLE FLOW TOOL

Flow Tool 7: Family Flow Map

GRANDPARENT GENERATION

	CONDITION	AGE AT ONSET	NOTES
Father's father			
Father's mother			
Mother's father			
Mother's mother			

TIP Flag a heart attack or stroke before age 55 in a male first-degree relative or before age 65 in a female first-degree relative. Write "unknown" if needed. Use another copy if you need more rows.

Look for patterns, not perfection.

PRINTABLE FLOW TOOL

Flow Tool 8: The 90-Day Flow Dashboard

PRINTABLE VERSION

Track only what you and your clinician decide is useful.

> Choose a few measures that can guide a decision. Your plan may change as recovery and treatment change.

METRIC	STARTING POINT	MY AGREED GOAL OR PLAN	REVIEW
Symptoms / function			
Blood pressure			
Lipid or other lab			
Movement / rehab			
Sleep / apnea plan			
Medication routine			
Follow-up			
Another measure			

flowheartandvascular.com/flow-tools

PRINTABLE FLOW TOOL

Flow Tool 8: The 90-Day Flow Dashboard

Track only what matters. Bring this dashboard to your review and ask what should stay, change, or stop.

Complete only what applies. Use clinician-set goals and review patterns, not isolated readings.

Review date: ______________________

What continues:

____

____

What changes:

____

____

What needs attention now:

____

____

Next review and what should happen before it:

____

____

____

PRINTABLE FLOW TOOL

Flow Tool 8: The 90-Day Flow Dashboard

Questions for the 90-Day Review

Medicine is not being taken consistently
Is the problem cost, side effects, confusion, schedule, access, or something else that can be solved?

Taken consistently, but the result remains off target
Does the dose, medicine, diagnosis, or goal need to change?

Side effects develop or a blood-test result becomes concerning
Does treatment need prompt adjustment, further testing, or a different option?

Symptoms persist despite an improved number
Have we treated a risk marker without explaining the symptom?

Function is declining
Does the diagnosis, rehabilitation plan, rhythm, heart function, anemia, lung disease, sleep, or mood need review?

> Set goals, safe ranges, and timing with your clinician. Follow any heart-failure daily-weight plan. Do not change medicines or activity limits based on this page alone. New, worsening, or severe symptoms should not wait for the review date.

PRINTABLE FLOW TOOL

Flow Tool 9: Questions Before a Planned Test or Procedure

PRINTABLE VERSION

These questions clarify what decision the test or procedure could change, its likely benefits and risks, and the alternatives.

Most cardiac tests and elective procedures are planned decisions. The right choice depends on what the test or procedure is expected to change. In a true emergency, follow emergency instructions first. For a nonemergency decision, bring these questions to the conversation before you agree to a planned test, stent, or procedure.

- What decision will this test or procedure help us make?
- Which question matters most here: what the heart or arteries look like, whether blood flow is limited, or what my overall risk is?
- What benefit should I realistically expect: relief of symptoms, prevention of an event, longer life, or better information?
- What risks matter most for me, given my kidney function, bleeding risk, allergies, frailty, medicines, and other conditions?
- What are the reasonable alternatives, including medical treatment, a different test, watchful waiting, or no immediate procedure?

flowheartandvascular.com/flow-tools

PRINTABLE FLOW TOOL

Flow Tool 9: Questions Before a Planned Test or Procedure

- What is likely to happen if I wait or decide not to proceed?
- Is this urgent, or is there time to discuss it further or obtain a second opinion?

> For a visible narrowing, ask whether it explains symptoms or limits blood flow, and which outcome the proposed treatment is expected to improve.

PRINTABLE FLOW TOOL

Flow Tool 10: My Cardiovascular Risk Snapshot: What I Can Change and What Changes the Goal

PRINTABLE VERSION

Fill in only the measures that apply to you, and leave the rest blank. Then set priorities with your clinician. This page is not a score or a diagnosis.

1. Blood Pressure

Recent readings: ______________________________

My clinician-set goal: ______________________________

Next step: ______________________________

2. Low-Density Lipoprotein Cholesterol (LDL-C) and Apolipoprotein B (ApoB): Treatable Plaque-Forming Risk

LDL-C or ApoB, if measured: ______________________________

My clinician-set LDL-C goal and ApoB goal, if used: __________

Next step: ______________________________

flowheartandvascular.com/flow-tools

Flow Tool 10: My Cardiovascular Risk Snapshot: What I Can Change and What Changes the Goal

3. Blood Sugar and Diabetes Risk

Hemoglobin A1c, an estimate of average blood sugar over about three months, or fasting glucose: ____________

My clinician-set goal: ____________

Next step: ____________

4. Smoking, Tobacco, and Vaping

Where I stand: ____________

My quit or stay-quit plan: ____________

5. Movement and Functional Fitness

Current activity, mobility, or function: ____________

My next safe, repeatable step: ____________

Sleep, Stress, and Support

Typical sleep: ____________ hours

Sleep-apnea assessment or treatment, if applicable: ____________

One practical support: ____________

PRINTABLE FLOW TOOL

Flow Tool 10: My Cardiovascular Risk Snapshot: What I Can Change and What Changes the Goal

Context That Can Change the Goal

This tool tracks factors that can be modified, but it is not a complete risk calculator. Also review the medical and family-history context that may change treatment targets:

- ☐ Established coronary artery disease, ischemic stroke or transient ischemic attack, aortic atherosclerosis, or peripheral artery disease
- ☐ Coronary plaque or calcium on imaging
- ☐ Chronic kidney disease
- ☐ Strong family history or familial hypercholesterolemia

Lipoprotein(a), or Lp(a), if measured:

________________________ nmol/L or mg/dL

How this result changes my LDL-C or prevention plan:

____

> Lp(a) is mostly inherited and usually does not fall meaningfully with lifestyle change. Its main role is to help determine how intensively LDL-C, ApoB, and other treatable risks should be managed.

____

PRINTABLE FLOW TOOL

Flow Tool 10: My Cardiovascular Risk Snapshot: What I Can Change and What Changes the Goal

- ☐ Pregnancy complications or menopause before age 40
- ☐ Autoimmune or chronic inflammatory disease
- ☐ Prior chest radiation or cancer treatment that can affect the heart or blood vessels

Use Flow Tool 7, Family Flow Map, for family history and Flow Tool 5, Women's and Pregnancy-Related Cardiovascular History Guide, for sex-specific history.

Work with your clinician to begin with the modifiable risk factor most likely to matter now. Then choose one change you can repeat.

PRINTABLE FLOW TOOL

Flow Tool 11: Symptom and Trend Tracker

PRINTABLE VERSION

Use one entry per symptom episode; use another sheet if several episodes occur in one day. Record the details when they occur rather than trying to reconstruct them later.

> Stop completing the tracker if symptoms are happening now or their pattern has changed. If any emergency feature is present, call 911; do not delay to finish the form. A low score from 0 to 10, or improvement with rest or nitroglycerin, does not prove that a symptom is safe.

Seven-Entry Symptom and Trend Log

Entry 1

Date and time: ______________

Symptom and severity, 0 to 10: ______________

Trigger, duration, and what relieved it: ______________

Blood pressure or heart rate, only if instructed: ______________

Action taken: ______________

Prescribed rescue medicine taken and response, if applicable:

PRINTABLE FLOW TOOL

Flow Tool 11: Symptom and Trend Tracker

Entry 2

Date and time: ______________________

Symptom and severity, 0 to 10: ______________________

Trigger, duration, and what relieved it: ______________________

Blood pressure or heart rate, only if instructed: ______________________

Action taken: ______________________

Prescribed rescue medicine taken and response, if applicable:

Entry 3

Date and time: ______________________

Symptom and severity, 0 to 10: ______________________

Trigger, duration, and what relieved it: ______________________

Blood pressure or heart rate, only if instructed: ______________________

Action taken: ______________________

Prescribed rescue medicine taken and response, if applicable:

PRINTABLE FLOW TOOL

Flow Tool 11: Symptom and Trend Tracker

Entry 4

Date and time: ______________________________

Symptom and severity, 0 to 10: ____________________

Trigger, duration, and what relieved it: ______________

Blood pressure or heart rate, only if instructed: _________

Action taken: ________________________________

Prescribed rescue medicine taken and response, if applicable:

Entry 5

Date and time: ______________________________

Symptom and severity, 0 to 10: ____________________

Trigger, duration, and what relieved it: ______________

Blood pressure or heart rate, only if instructed: _________

Action taken: ________________________________

Prescribed rescue medicine taken and response, if applicable:

PRINTABLE FLOW TOOL

Flow Tool 11: Symptom and Trend Tracker

Entry 6

Date and time: ____________________

Symptom and severity, 0 to 10: ____________________

Trigger, duration, and what relieved it: ____________________

Blood pressure or heart rate, only if instructed: ____________________

Action taken: ____________________

Prescribed rescue medicine taken and response, if applicable:

Entry 7

Date and time: ____________________

Symptom and severity, 0 to 10: ____________________

Trigger, duration, and what relieved it: ____________________

Blood pressure or heart rate, only if instructed: ____________________

Action taken: ____________________

Prescribed rescue medicine taken and response, if applicable:

Bring this page to your appointment. Include how long each symptom lasted and whether it stopped with rest or prescribed medicine.

PRINTABLE FLOW TOOL

Flow Tool 12: Flow Maintenance Checklist Beyond 90 Days

PRINTABLE VERSION

Use this page at the interval you and your clinician choose. Long-term follow-up depends on diagnoses, medicines, recent events, and symptoms.

Symptoms and Function

- ☐ New or changing chest discomfort, breathlessness, palpitations, faintness, swelling, fatigue, or exercise limitation reviewed
- ☐ Daily function, work, driving, intimacy, and activity concerns discussed when relevant
- ☐ Emergency and same-day call instructions still understood

Medicines

- ☐ Medication list reconciled with what I actually take
- ☐ Purpose and intended duration of each medicine reviewed
- ☐ Side effects, cost, refills, missed doses, and access problems discussed
- ☐ Sick-day and procedure instructions recorded when needed
- ☐ Over-the-counter medicines and supplements reviewed for interactions

flowheartandvascular.com/flow-tools

PRINTABLE FLOW TOOL

Flow Tool 12: Flow Maintenance Checklist Beyond 90 Days

Measurements and Monitoring

- [ ] Home blood-pressure average reviewed if monitoring was assigned
- [ ] Lipid testing completed when due
- [ ] Kidney function and blood salts such as sodium and potassium checked for medicines or conditions that require them
- [ ] If applicable, A1c or another blood sugar measure reviewed along with related heart, kidney, or metabolic conditions
- [ ] Heart-failure weight or fluid plan reviewed if applicable

Recovery and Prevention

- [ ] Support and treatment for stopping tobacco or nicotine use reviewed if applicable
- [ ] Cardiac rehabilitation, activity, strength, balance, or fall concerns reviewed
- [ ] Sleep-apnea evaluation or treatment reviewed if applicable
- [ ] Mood, anxiety, trauma symptoms, and social support discussed
- [ ] Nutrition goals fit my diagnoses, culture, preferences, and access to food

PRINTABLE FLOW TOOL

Flow Tool 12: Flow Maintenance Checklist Beyond 90 Days

Closing the Loop

- ☐ I know who will review each pending referral, test, or result
- ☐ I understand why repeat imaging is planned and how the result could change care
- ☐ Next review date is written down
- ☐ I know which change should prompt an earlier call

What continues: ____________________

What changes: ____________________

Next review date: ____________________

> If symptoms are new or worsening, do not wait for the next scheduled review. If an emergency feature is present, call 911; otherwise contact your clinician promptly.

PRINTABLE FLOW TOOL

Flow Tool 13: A Quick Guide for Family and Caregivers

PRINTABLE VERSION

How to support someone protecting their heart without taking over.

If someone you love is working to protect their heart, ask what kind of help they want. Some people welcome reminders or company; others do not. Agree on your role instead of assuming it.

- Ask how you can help instead of assigning tasks.
- Offer to walk, prepare meals, or adjust routines together.
- Learn the emergency warning signs together, and never discourage someone from calling for help.
- If side effects occur, help them contact the prescribing team rather than stopping a medicine.
- Review your own cardiovascular risk factors, especially when conditions run in the family.

> Caregiving can affect your sleep, mood, health, and ability to function. Ask the clinical team or your own clinician for support when caregiving is affecting your well-being or becoming difficult to manage safely.

flowheartandvascular.com/flow-tools

PRINTABLE FLOW TOOL

Flow Tool 14: If Your Watch Flags Possible AFib

PRINTABLE VERSION

If your watch flags possible atrial fibrillation (AFib), save what it recorded and check how you feel before deciding what to do next.

First: Check for Emergency Symptoms

Call 911 for stroke signs, severe chest pressure, fainting, severe breathlessness, or a fast or irregular heartbeat with dizziness or near-fainting. Do not drive yourself.

If You Feel Well

- Save the tracing or screenshot if your device recorded one.
- Write down the time, how long the alert lasted, any symptoms, what you were doing, and anything unusual such as illness, dehydration, poor sleep, or alcohol.
- Contact your clinician so the rhythm can be reviewed and, when appropriate, confirmed with an electrocardiogram (ECG) or medical monitor.
- Keep taking prescribed medicines unless the prescribing team tells you otherwise.

flowheartandvascular.com/flow-tools

PRINTABLE FLOW TOOL

Flow Tool 14: If Your Watch Flags Possible AFib

Wearable Alert Rule

An isolated alert without emergency symptoms is not, by itself, proof of AFib. Arrange prompt clinical review and do not self-treat. Repeated alerts, a sustained fast or irregular rhythm, new symptoms, or a worsening pattern warrant same-day contact with your clinician; use the emergency instructions above if severe symptoms develop.

A wearable alert is not a confirmed diagnosis, and the absence of an alert does not rule out AFib. Save the tracing when possible. Do not start aspirin or an anticoagulant, take extra heart-rate medicine, or change another prescription based on a watch alert alone.

Flow Glossary

Use this glossary to understand what a term means and why it matters. Where confusion is common, it also explains what the term does not mean and points you to related terms.

A

A1c (hemoglobin A1c): a blood test that estimates your average blood sugar over the past two to three months.
Why it matters: A1c reflects blood sugar over time and can reveal persistent elevation that one fasting value may miss.

Ablation: a procedure that uses catheters to target heart tissue involved in an abnormal rhythm. In AFib, the usual goal is to reduce recurrent arrhythmia and symptoms. (Chapter 9)
Why it matters: Ablation can improve rhythm control in selected patients, but success rates and procedural risks depend on the rhythm, heart structure, other conditions, and prior treatment.
What it does not mean: Successful ablation does not automatically remove the need for anticoagulation. Stroke prevention remains based on the patient's risk and current clinical guidance.
See also: *Atrial fibrillation; Cardioversion; Anticoagulants.*

Absolute risk, relative risk, and absolute risk reduction: absolute risk is the chance that an event will occur in a defined group over a defined period. Relative risk compares the event rate between groups. Absolute risk reduction is the difference between those event rates.
Why it matters: A treatment can produce the same relative reduction but a larger absolute benefit in a person whose starting risk is higher. Ask about absolute effects when they are available.
What it does not mean: A group average cannot predict exactly what will happen to one person.

ACE inhibitor / ARB / ARNI: related medication groups that relax blood vessels or alter hormone signals. ACE stands for angiotensin-converting enzyme; ARB for angiotensin receptor blocker; and ARNI for angiotensin receptor–neprilysin inhibitor. They are used for specific blood-pressure, heart-failure, kidney, and post-heart-attack indications. (Chapter 14)

Why it matters: Benefits depend on the indication. These medicines require monitoring of blood pressure, kidney function, potassium, and drug-specific side effects. ACE inhibitors, ARBs, and ARNIs are not used during pregnancy.

Acute coronary syndrome (ACS): an urgent condition caused by suddenly reduced blood flow to heart muscle. It includes unstable angina and heart attack.

Why it matters: New, severe, worsening, persistent, or resting chest discomfort may represent ACS and needs urgent evaluation. Call 911 when symptoms may be an emergency.

See also: *Heart attack (myocardial infarction); Stable versus unstable angina; STEMI; NSTEMI.*

Adverse pregnancy outcome: a pregnancy complication associated with higher later cardiovascular risk, including preeclampsia, gestational hypertension, gestational diabetes, and preterm delivery. (Chapter 5)

Why it matters: Pregnancy history can reveal susceptibility years before traditional risk factors become obvious. It should be included in long-term cardiovascular history and may support earlier review of blood pressure, glucose, lipids, weight, and other risks.

What it does not mean: A complication does not mean that cardiovascular disease is inevitable or that every woman needs the same test or medicine.

Angina: chest discomfort or another symptom caused when heart muscle temporarily does not receive enough blood and oxygen. It may feel like pressure, breathlessness, or unusual fatigue with activity. Clinicians call the underlying problem ischemia. (Chapter 8)
Why it matters: Angina is one way ischemia can be felt. Ischemia can also be silent, and similar symptoms can have noncardiac causes.

ANOCA: angina with nonobstructive coronary arteries: symptoms consistent with angina even though no major coronary blockage is found. It describes the clinical presentation; the cause still requires evaluation. (Chapter 11)
Why it matters: Possible causes include problems in the heart's smallest vessels, coronary spasm, plaque spread throughout the arteries, or a noncardiac condition.

Angiogram (invasive): an imaging test that uses contrast dye to outline the open channel inside your coronary arteries.
What it does not mean: A "clean" angiogram does not rule out plaque in the artery wall or disease in the smallest vessels.
See also: *Cardiac catheterization; FFR / iFR; Coronary CT angiogram (CCTA).*

Anticoagulants (including direct oral anticoagulants and warfarin): medicines used for atrial fibrillation, clots in a deep vein or the lungs (venous thromboembolism), mechanical heart valves, and other specific conditions. For anyone with a mechanical heart valve, and for people with AFib who have rheumatic mitral stenosis or mitral stenosis of moderate or greater severity, warfarin is generally used rather than a direct oral anticoagulant. (Chapters 9 and 14)
Why it matters: Anticoagulants are not interchangeable with antiplatelets or automatically with one another. The indication, dose, kidney function, bleeding risk, interactions, and valve type matter.
See also: *Dual antiplatelet therapy (DAPT); Atrial fibrillation (AFib).*

Antiplatelet medicine: a drug that reduces the ability of platelets to form a clot. Aspirin and P2Y12 inhibitors such as clopidogrel, prasugrel, and ticagrelor are common examples. (Chapter 14)

Why it matters: Antiplatelet treatment is used for specific artery problems, especially after many heart attacks, unstable coronary events, and stent procedures. The medicine combination and duration depend on the risks of inadequate blood flow, clotting, and bleeding.

What it does not mean: Antiplatelets are not interchangeable with anticoagulants. Do not stop a prescribed antiplatelet after a recent stent without direct guidance from the cardiology team.

See also: *Dual antiplatelet therapy (DAPT); Anticoagulants; Stent.*

ApoB (Apolipoprotein B): a measure of how many potentially plaque-forming lipoprotein particles are circulating in the blood.

Why it matters: ApoB can add useful risk information when the LDL-C value and the number of particles tell different stories, especially with diabetes, high triglycerides, or metabolic disease.

See also: *LDL-C (low-density lipoprotein cholesterol); Lipoprotein(a), or Lp(a); Statin; PCSK9-directed therapy.*

Arrhythmia: an abnormal heart rhythm that is too fast, too slow, or irregular.

Why it matters: Rhythm problems and artery problems are different issues; one does not automatically mean the other.

What it does not mean: It does not by itself mean you are having or about to have a heart attack.

ASCVD (atherosclerotic cardiovascular disease): disease caused by plaque in the arteries, including coronary heart disease, many ischemic strokes, and peripheral artery disease.
Why it matters: Once ASCVD is established, treatment is considered secondary prevention. The diagnosis usually supports more intensive risk reduction than primary prevention in a person who has not had clinical atherosclerotic disease.
What it does not mean: ASCVD does not include every cause of heart disease or stroke. Rhythm disorders, valve disease, heart-muscle disease, hemorrhagic stroke, and nonatherosclerotic vascular disorders require their own assessment.

Atherosclerosis: the underlying disease process in which plaque builds up within the artery wall over years.
Why it matters: Atherosclerosis is a major cause of heart attack, ischemic stroke, and peripheral artery disease, although each condition also has other causes. It can develop long before symptoms appear.

Atrial fibrillation (AFib): a common irregular heart rhythm originating in the heart's upper chambers. (Chapter 9)
Why it matters: AFib can raise stroke risk and can affect symptoms or heart function, but it is a rhythm problem distinct from blocked arteries. Stroke prevention and rate-or-rhythm treatment are separate decisions. A wearable alert is not a confirmed diagnosis.

B

Bempedoic acid: an oral nonstatin medicine that lowers LDL-C by reducing cholesterol synthesis in the liver. (Chapter 14)
Why it matters: It can reduce cardiovascular events in selected statin-intolerant, high-risk patients and may be used alone or with other lipid-lowering treatment.
What it does not mean: It is not free of adverse effects or appropriate for every patient who reports muscle symptoms. Elevated uric acid or gout, tendon problems, drug interactions, expected LDL-C reduction, and overall risk may affect the choice.
See also: *Statin; Ezetimibe; PCSK9-directed therapy.*

Beta blocker: a medication that slows heart rate, reduces oxygen demand, and stabilizes rhythm. (Chapter 14)
Why it matters: Beta blockers are important for selected conditions, including heart failure with reduced pumping strength, angina, rhythm disorders, high blood pressure, and some patients after a heart attack. Long-term need depends on why the medicine was prescribed, pumping strength, symptoms, rhythm, and current evidence.

Blood pressure (BP): the force of blood against artery walls with every heartbeat.
Why it matters: Sustained high blood pressure raises the risk of heart attack, stroke, heart failure, kidney disease, and other complications. Repeated measurements show the pattern better than one reading.

C

CABG (coronary artery bypass grafting, or bypass surgery): an operation that uses one or more grafts to route blood around one or more narrowed or blocked coronary arteries. (Chapter 13)
Why it matters: CABG can improve symptoms. For some patients, it can also improve long-term outcomes, depending on which arteries are affected, how complex the disease is, and the patient's overall condition. Medicines and risk-factor treatment remain important afterward.
See also: *Stent; Revascularization; PCI.*

Coronary artery calcium (CAC) score: a CT scan that measures calcified plaque already present in your coronary arteries.
Why it matters: The amount and distribution of coronary calcium can refine long-term risk and help guide prevention in an appropriate adult without symptoms. In selected low-risk patients with stable chest pain, CAC may also be used as a first-line test for calcified plaque.
What it does not mean: A score of zero does not prove there is no noncalcified plaque, and a high score does not automatically mean you need a stent.

Cardiac arrest: the sudden loss of effective blood pumping by the heart, usually because of a dangerous disturbance in its electrical rhythm. The person collapses, becomes unresponsive, and is not breathing normally or is only gasping. (Chapter 1)
Why it matters: Cardiac arrest is a medical emergency. Call 911, begin cardiopulmonary resuscitation (CPR), and use an automated external defibrillator (AED) as soon as one is available. A heart attack can trigger cardiac arrest, but most heart attacks do not, and cardiac arrest can have other causes.
See also: *Heart attack (myocardial infarction); Arrhythmia.*

Cardiac catheterization ("cath"): a procedure in which a thin tube is passed through a blood vessel to the heart, usually to measure pressures, take pictures of the coronary arteries (an angiogram), or sometimes treat a blockage.
Why it matters: It lets clinicians see a blockage and, when appropriate, treat it, but seeing a narrowing is not the same as proving it needs treatment.
See also: *Angiogram (invasive); Stent; FFR / iFR.*

Cardiac rehabilitation: a structured program of supervised exercise, education, risk-factor management, and support after selected heart events or procedures. (Chapter 15)
Why it matters: Cardiac rehabilitation can improve function and quality of life and reduce hospitalizations. Ask about home-based or hybrid options if attendance is difficult.

Cardioversion: treatment that attempts to restore a normal rhythm using a controlled electrical shock or selected medicine. (Chapter 9)
Why it matters: Cardioversion can relieve symptoms and restore rhythm in selected patients with AFib or another arrhythmia. Timing, anticoagulation, imaging, and recurrence risk require planning.
What it does not mean: Restoring rhythm does not prove that AFib will not return and does not by itself remove stroke risk.
See also: *Atrial fibrillation; Ablation; Anticoagulants.*

Cascade screening: the practice of testing relatives step by step after one person is diagnosed with an inherited condition such as familial hypercholesterolemia. (Chapter 6)
Why it matters: Parents, siblings, and children may benefit from earlier evaluation and treatment. Children should receive age-appropriate testing through their clinician rather than waiting until adulthood.
What it does not mean: Cascade screening does not mean that every relative inherited the condition or will have the same degree of risk. Testing should be specific to the condition and voluntary.
See also: *Familial hypercholesterolemia (FH); Lipoprotein(a), or Lp(a); Variant of uncertain significance (VUS).*

Chest pressure vs. chest pain: heart-related discomfort can take either form. It is not always the dramatic, crushing pain people expect.
Why it matters: Many people describe pressure, heaviness, tightness, or even indigestion-like discomfort. Dismissing it because it isn't sharp "pain" is a common and dangerous mistake.

Clot (thrombus): a mass of blood cells, platelets, and clotting proteins that forms within a blood vessel or heart chamber. Clots can arise for different reasons, including plaque breaking open, blood moving too slowly or sitting relatively still (stasis), or injury to a vein. (Chapters 2 and 9)
Why it matters: A coronary clot can sharply reduce blood flow during a heart attack or unstable coronary event; a clot in a vein or heart chamber can travel to the lungs or brain. Treatment depends on the setting and must balance expected benefit with bleeding risk.

Continuous positive airway pressure (CPAP): treatment that uses gentle air pressure through a mask to keep the upper airway open during sleep. (Chapter 7)
Why it matters: CPAP can reduce breathing interruptions and improve sleepiness and quality of life; it may modestly lower blood pressure. It should not be promised to prevent a heart attack or stroke.

Coronary computed tomography angiography (CCTA): a CT scan using intravenous contrast dye to show coronary plaque, its location, whether it is calcified or noncalcified, and the degree of narrowing.
Why it matters: Unlike a stress test, it can see disease before it limits blood flow.

What it does not mean: A normal CCTA is reassuring but reflects one moment in time; it does not guarantee plaque will stay stable in the future.

Coronary flow reserve (CFR): the ratio of coronary blood flow during stress to flow at rest. (Chapter 11)
Why it matters: A low CFR can result from a major blockage, plaque spread throughout the arteries, or problems in the heart's smallest vessels. After significant large-vessel disease has been excluded or accounted for, it can support a small-vessel diagnosis.

Coronary spasm: a temporary tightening of a coronary artery that reduces blood flow and can cause chest discomfort or ischemia even when no fixed major narrowing is present. (Chapter 11)
Why it matters: It often strikes at rest, in the early morning, or in the cold rather than during exertion, and it responds to a different set of medications than fixed plaque.
See also: *Ischemia; Microvascular dysfunction, coronary.*

D

Diabetes / prediabetes: Diabetes is a condition in which blood sugar stays too high because the body does not make enough insulin, does not use insulin properly, or both. Prediabetes means blood-sugar levels are above the usual range but below the diabetes threshold; progression is not inevitable.
Why it matters: Prediabetes raises the chance of developing diabetes and often occurs alongside other cardiovascular risks, including excess abdominal fat, abnormal cholesterol, and high blood pressure.

Dual antiplatelet therapy (DAPT): a combination of aspirin and a second antiplatelet drug, used especially after a stent. (Chapter 14)
What it does not mean: Do not stop DAPT after a stent without guidance from the prescribing cardiology team; stopping too early can cause a dangerous clot inside the stent (stent thrombosis), while continuing longer than needed can increase bleeding.

E

Ejection fraction (EF): the percentage of blood in the heart's main pumping chamber that is pumped out with each beat. (Chapter 8)
What it does not mean: A normal EF does not by itself rule out heart failure or other heart disease.

Electrocardiogram (ECG): a test that records the heart's electrical activity through electrodes placed on the skin.
Why it matters: It can show rhythm problems and some signs of current or prior heart injury.
What it does not mean: A normal ECG does not by itself rule out a heart attack, reduced blood flow, or other heart disease.

Endothelium: the one-cell-thick lining of every blood vessel in your body. (Chapter 2)
Why it matters: A well-functioning endothelium helps vessels widen and regulates inflammation, clotting, and healing. Dysfunction can contribute to atherosclerosis and problems regulating blood flow.
See also: *Plaque; Microvascular dysfunction, coronary.*

Ezetimibe: an oral medicine that lowers LDL-C by reducing intestinal cholesterol absorption; it may be used alone or with a statin. (Chapter 14)
Why it matters: It is one evidence-based option when additional LDL lowering is needed or a statin is not tolerated at the desired dose.
See also: *Statin; LDL-C (low-density lipoprotein cholesterol); ApoB (Apolipoprotein B); Bempedoic acid; PCSK9-directed therapy.*

F

Familial hypercholesterolemia (FH): an inherited condition that causes very high LDL cholesterol from early life. Lifestyle remains important, but lifestyle alone generally does not explain or correct the degree of LDL elevation.
Why it matters: Because it runs in families, one person's diagnosis is a reason to offer family-based testing to parents, siblings, and children. Earlier identification can allow treatment decades sooner.
See also: *LDL-C; Lipoprotein(a), or Lp(a); Statin; PCSK9-directed therapy.*

FFR / iFR: fractional flow reserve (FFR) and instantaneous wave-free ratio (iFR) are pressure-based measurements used during coronary angiography to estimate whether a specific narrowing is likely to limit blood flow. (Chapters 12 and 13)
Why it matters: They add information about whether a narrowing is actually restricting blood flow, but they do not directly show whether plaque is likely to break open or how the smallest vessels function.

Fibrous cap: a layer of fibrous tissue that covers a plaque and separates its contents from the bloodstream. (Chapter 2)
Why it matters: A thin or disrupted cap is one feature associated with plaque rupture. Risk also reflects plaque burden, inflammation, narrowing, and the patient's overall clinical context.

Flow: this book's teaching framework for connecting what is present in the heart and arteries, what it is doing to blood flow and function, and what it means for the patient over time. (Chapter 3)
Why it matters: It can help patients ask clearer questions. It is not a diagnosis, risk calculator, or substitute for established clinical terms.

Flow Engine: this book's name for the connected biology of the endothelium, artery wall, and microcirculation. It is one part of the broader Flow framework. (Chapter 3)
Why it matters: It reminds readers that an artery is a living system and that anatomy, blood-flow function, and risk are related but not interchangeable questions.

G

GLP-1 receptor agonists and dual GIP/GLP-1 medicines: medicines used for specific diabetes and chronic weight-management indications. Evidence about cardiovascular outcomes and approved uses differs by medicine; several GLP-1 receptor agonists reduce cardiovascular events in defined groups. (Chapter 14)

Why it matters: Expected benefits vary by medicine and indication and may include glucose control, weight loss, kidney benefit, or fewer cardiovascular events.

What it does not mean: A GLP-1 medicine may be one part of the plan. It does not replace other indicated treatment.

H

HDL-C (high-density lipoprotein cholesterol): the amount of cholesterol carried in HDL particles.

Why it matters: HDL-C contributes to risk assessment, but it is not a treatment target in the same way as LDL-C or ApoB. Medicines that raise HDL-C have not reliably reduced cardiovascular events.

What it does not mean: A high HDL-C does not cancel the risk associated with high LDL-C, ApoB, smoking, diabetes, high blood pressure, or established plaque.

See also: *LDL-C; ApoB (Apolipoprotein B).*

Heart attack (myocardial infarction): injury to heart muscle caused by a sudden lack of blood and oxygen, often when plaque breaks open or erodes and a clot sharply reduces or blocks blood flow in a coronary artery.

Why it matters: Some heart attacks follow years of atherosclerosis; others have different causes, including a tear in an artery wall, spasm, a clot that travels from elsewhere, or another major strain that makes the heart need more oxygen than the blood can supply.

See also: *Plaque rupture; Clot (thrombus); STEMI; NSTEMI.*

Heart failure: a clinical syndrome in which a structural or functional heart abnormality causes symptoms or signs. The heart may squeeze weakly or may fill only at abnormally high pressure. It can cause breathlessness, fatigue, swelling, or reduced ability to be active. (Chapter 8)

Why it matters: It has many causes and several forms, and treatment can improve symptoms, hospitalization risk, and survival.

Heart Team: a multidisciplinary group that jointly evaluates complex coronary decisions. It typically includes an interventional cardiologist, a cardiac surgeon, and other specialists as needed. (Chapter 13)

Why it matters: When the best revascularization strategy is uncertain, such as in significant left-main disease or complex disease in several arteries, a Heart Team discussion compares PCI with bypass surgery and weighs durability, recovery, procedural risk, diabetes, heart function, anatomy, and what matters most to the patient.

What it does not mean: A Heart Team recommendation does not replace the patient's decision or automatically mean that a procedure is needed.

See also: *PCI (percutaneous coronary intervention); CABG (coronary artery bypass grafting); Revascularization.*

HFpEF / HFmrEF / HFrEF: abbreviations you may see in a report for heart failure with preserved, mildly reduced, or reduced pumping strength. The categories are based partly on ejection fraction, the percentage of blood pumped from the heart's main chamber with each beat. (Chapter 8)

Why it matters: Ejection fraction helps guide treatment, but symptoms, whether pressure is backing up, the heart's structure, and the cause are also needed to understand the condition.

hs-CRP: high-sensitivity C-reactive protein, a blood test that can detect low levels of general inflammation in the body; it does not identify the source. (Chapter 12)
Why it matters: A persistent elevation may add risk information in selected patients, but infection, injury, autoimmune disease, and many other conditions can raise it. It does not measure inflammation inside a specific plaque.

I

INOCA (ischemia with nonobstructive coronary arteries): objective evidence that heart muscle is not receiving enough blood for its workload even though the large coronary arteries do not have a major flow-limiting blockage. Symptoms without documented ischemia are often described as ANOCA, angina with nonobstructive coronary arteries. (Chapters 5 and 11)
Why it matters: Possible causes include problems in the heart's smallest vessels, spasm of a large or small coronary artery, plaque spread throughout the arteries, or more than one mechanism. The cause can influence testing and treatment.
What it does not mean: INOCA is not a synonym for coronary microvascular dysfunction, and a normal angiogram alone does not establish the diagnosis.
See also: *Microvascular dysfunction, coronary; Coronary spasm; MINOCA.*

Insulin resistance: a condition in which the body does not respond normally to insulin, so more insulin is often needed to keep blood sugar in range. Over time, blood sugar may rise.
Why it matters: Insulin resistance often occurs with prediabetes or type 2 diabetes and can accompany high triglycerides, visceral fat, fatty liver disease, and other cardiovascular risks.
See also: *Diabetes / prediabetes; Visceral fat.*

Ischemia: too little oxygen-rich blood reaching heart muscle for the amount of work it is doing. (Chapter 8)
Why it matters: Ischemia may result from a major plaque-related narrowing, spasm, problems in the heart's smallest vessels, anemia, a rapid rhythm, or other causes. It can cause angina or be silent.

L

LDL-C (low-density lipoprotein cholesterol): the amount of cholesterol carried in LDL particles, which are causally involved in atherosclerosis.
Why it matters: Lowering LDL-C reduces cardiovascular events. The treatment goal depends on baseline risk, established disease, plaque burden, and current guidelines.
What it does not mean: An LDL in the "normal range" on a lab report is not the same as an optimal LDL for your level of risk.
See also: *ApoB (Apolipoprotein B); Lipoprotein(a), or Lp(a); HDL-C.*

Left atrial appendage: a small pouch attached to the left upper chamber of the heart. (Chapter 9)
Why it matters: In atrial fibrillation, blood can pool in this pouch and form a clot that may travel to the brain and cause a stroke. For selected patients at elevated stroke risk who have a strong reason not to take long-term anticoagulation, a procedure that seals the appendage may be considered.
What it does not mean: Closing the appendage does not treat AFib, eliminate every source of stroke, or automatically replace anticoagulation for everyone.
See also: *Atrial fibrillation (AFib); Anticoagulants (including direct oral anticoagulants and warfarin).*

Lipoprotein(a), or Lp(a): a mostly inherited cholesterol-related particle associated with plaque-related artery disease and calcium-related narrowing of the aortic valve.
Why it matters: Lp(a) level is largely genetically determined and changes little with lifestyle. Current guidance recommends at least one adult measurement; a high result may support more intensive management of other modifiable risks.
See also: *LDL-C (low-density lipoprotein cholesterol); ApoB (Apolipoprotein B); Atherosclerosis.*

M

Microcirculation: the network of the heart's smallest blood vessels, which helps match blood flow to the heart muscle's changing needs. (Chapters 3 and 11)
Why it matters: Problems in this network can cause symptoms or reduced blood flow even when the large coronary arteries do not have a major blockage.

Microvascular dysfunction, coronary: a problem in which the heart's smallest blood vessels do not widen or control blood flow normally. It may occur in women or men and requires clinical assessment and, when appropriate, dedicated testing. (Chapters 5 and 11)
Why it matters: It is one possible cause of ischemia or angina without a major coronary blockage. A routine angiogram does not directly show the smallest vessels. Specialized testing during a heart catheterization can evaluate how these vessels respond, and selected scans can measure blood flow to the heart and how much it increases under stress.
What it does not mean: Symptoms plus a normal angiogram do not prove coronary microvascular dysfunction. A major blockage, coronary spasm, rhythm disorders, structural heart disease, lung disease, digestive causes, muscle or joint pain, anemia, and other explanations may still need consideration.
See also: *INOCA; Coronary spasm; Coronary flow reserve.*

MINOCA (myocardial infarction with nonobstructive coronary arteries): a starting diagnosis used when testing confirms a heart attack but an angiogram does not show a major blocked coronary artery that explains it. Further testing is needed to identify the cause. (Chapter 5)
Why it matters: Possible causes include plaque breaking open, coronary spasm, SCAD, a clot that traveled into a coronary artery, and problems in the heart's smallest vessels. Cardiac MRI and other testing may reveal heart-muscle inflammation or Takotsubo syndrome, which are not heart attacks and require a different diagnosis.
What it does not mean: MINOCA does not mean a mild or imaginary heart attack. It also does not identify the mechanism by itself.
See also: *Heart attack (myocardial infarction); SCAD; Takotsubo syndrome; Coronary spasm.*

Myocardial injury: a finding that cardiac troponin is above the assay's 99th-percentile upper reference limit, indicating injury to heart muscle. A rising or falling pattern supports recent injury; a stable elevation may reflect long-standing injury. (Chapter 8)
Why it matters: Myocardial injury is a finding, not a cause. Heart failure, a rapid rhythm, myocarditis, a lung clot, kidney disease, plaque-related ischemia, and other conditions can raise troponin; the clinical context determines the diagnosis.
What it does not mean: An elevated troponin does not automatically mean a heart attack or that a plaque has ruptured. Heart attack (myocardial infarction) requires recent myocardial injury plus clinical evidence that inadequate blood flow caused it.
See also: *Troponin; Heart attack (myocardial infarction); Ischemia.*

N

Natriuretic peptides (BNP / NT-proBNP): blood tests that can rise when the heart is under strain or pressures inside the heart are elevated. (Chapter 8)

Why it matters: These markers help support a diagnosis of heart failure when combined with symptoms, examination, and imaging, especially when ejection fraction is not clearly reduced. Levels must be interpreted with age, kidney function, atrial fibrillation, obesity, and other factors.

What it does not mean: An elevated value alone does not diagnose heart failure or determine its cause, and a normal value does not completely exclude it in every setting. BNP and NT-proBNP values are not interchangeable.

See also: *Heart failure; Ejection fraction (EF); HFpEF / HFmrEF / HFrEF.*

Nitrates (including nitroglycerin): medicines that relax blood vessels and can relieve angina; short-acting nitroglycerin is often prescribed as a rescue medicine for episodes of chest discomfort. (Chapter 11 and Toolkit)

Why it matters: Nitrates can help symptoms in selected patients, including some with coronary spasm. Critical safety rule: never combine nitrates with erectile-dysfunction medicines such as sildenafil or tadalafil; the combination can cause a dangerous drop in blood pressure.

What it does not mean: Relief after nitroglycerin does not prove that discomfort came from the heart. Taking it is not a substitute for calling 911 when symptoms may represent a heart attack or another emergency.

See also: *Angina; Coronary spasm; Stable versus unstable angina.*

Nonobstructive coronary arteries and nonobstructive plaque: "Nonobstructive coronary arteries" means that no major coronary artery has a narrowing at or above the usual obstructive threshold, commonly 50%. It does not by itself say whether plaque is absent. CCTA may show no plaque or plaque below that threshold, whereas invasive angiography outlines the lumen and may not reveal plaque within the wall. Plaque present below the threshold is called nonobstructive coronary plaque or nonobstructive coronary artery disease. (Chapters 5 and 11)

Why it matters: Nonobstructive plaque is still coronary disease and can progress. Symptoms or ischemia can also occur without obstructive plaque because of diffuse disease, coronary spasm, or problems in the heart's smallest vessels.

What it does not mean: The label does not mean that symptoms are imaginary or that cardiovascular risk is zero. Exact wording and thresholds can vary by test and clinical setting.

See also: *ANOCA; INOCA (ischemia with nonobstructive coronary arteries); MINOCA (myocardial infarction with nonobstructive coronary arteries); Plaque; Coronary spasm.*

NSTEMI (non-ST-elevation myocardial infarction): a heart attack without the classic persistent ST-elevation pattern on the ECG. Diagnosis depends on the clinical picture, a rise or fall in troponin, and evidence that heart muscle was not receiving enough blood. It should not be defined simply as an incompletely blocked artery.

Why it matters: NSTEMI is a true heart attack. Its urgency and treatment depend on symptoms, ECG changes, stability, anatomy, and overall risk.

O

Obstructive sleep apnea (OSA): repeated narrowing or closure of the upper airway during sleep, causing fragmented sleep and often intermittent oxygen changes. (Chapter 7)

Why it matters: OSA is associated with hypertension, rhythm problems, daytime impairment, and cardiovascular disease. Treatment can improve breathing, sleepiness, quality of life, and blood pressure; it should not be promised to prevent a heart attack or stroke.

P

PCI (percutaneous coronary intervention): a catheter-based procedure used to open a coronary narrowing, usually with balloon dilation and placement of a stent. (Chapter 13)

Why it matters: PCI can restore blood flow urgently during selected acute coronary syndromes and can relieve angina from a flow-limiting narrowing in stable disease.

What it does not mean: PCI does not remove atherosclerosis from the rest of the arterial system or replace indicated medical therapy.

See also: *Stent; Revascularization; CABG; FFR/iFR.*

PCSK9-directed therapy: treatment that lowers LDL-C and ApoB by increasing the liver's ability to clear LDL particles. Injectable medicines such as evolocumab and alirocumab block PCSK9 in the blood; inclisiran uses a different approach to reduce the liver's production of PCSK9. (Chapter 14)

Why it matters: Evolocumab and alirocumab lower LDL and have demonstrated fewer cardiovascular events in selected high-risk patients. Inclisiran lowers LDL cholesterol, but whether it reduces cardiovascular events remains under study.

What it does not mean: These medicines are not interchangeable. They differ in how often they are given, which patients they are approved for, what their trials have shown, and what insurance will cover. Your clinician should choose one based on the job it needs to do for you.

See also: *Statin; Ezetimibe; Bempedoic acid; LDL-C; ApoB.*

Peripartum cardiomyopathy: heart failure caused by new weakening of the heart's main pumping chamber near the end of pregnancy or in the months after delivery when another cause is not found. (Chapter 5)
Why it matters: Breathlessness, swelling, fatigue, and difficulty lying flat can overlap with common pregnancy or postpartum symptoms. A new or severe pattern requires prompt evaluation.
What it does not mean: Ordinary postpartum fatigue or swelling does not prove cardiomyopathy. Diagnosis requires clinical assessment and cardiac testing.

Peripheral artery disease (PAD): atherosclerotic narrowing or blockage in arteries that carry blood to the legs or arms, most often the legs and feet.
Why it matters: PAD may cause leg discomfort with walking, slow-healing wounds, or threatened limb blood flow, and it raises the risk of heart attack and stroke even when leg symptoms are mild or absent.
What it does not mean: Leg pain alone does not establish PAD; examination and vascular testing may be needed.
See also: *ASCVD; Atherosclerosis.*

Positron emission tomography (PET) blood-flow imaging and stress cardiac magnetic resonance imaging (MRI): advanced scans that can examine blood flow to the heart without placing a catheter in an artery. PET can measure blood flow at rest and during stress. Stress cardiac MRI can examine blood flow, pumping function, and the heart muscle itself. (Chapter 11)
Why it matters: These tests may help when symptoms persist, obstructive disease does not explain them, or microvascular dysfunction is being considered.
What it does not mean: An abnormal flow reserve does not, by itself, prove a single cause. Availability and local expertise vary.

Plaque: a buildup of cholesterol-rich and inflammatory material within the artery wall.
Why it matters: Risk reflects total plaque burden, composition, inflammation, narrowing, location, and the patient's overall clinical context rather than size alone.

Plaque erosion: a mechanism in which the surface over a plaque becomes damaged without the fibrous cap breaking open, allowing a blood clot to form at that site and reduce blood flow. (Chapters 1–2)
Why it matters: Along with plaque rupture, erosion is one way a Type 1 heart attack can begin. The plaque may not have appeared severe beforehand, which helps explain why some events feel sudden.

What it does not mean: Not every plaque will erode or rupture, and no imaging test can reliably predict which individual plaque will cause trouble.

See also: *Plaque; Plaque rupture; Clot (thrombus); Type 1 and Type 2 myocardial infarction.*

Plaque rupture: a break in the fibrous cap covering a plaque that exposes plaque contents to the bloodstream and can trigger a clot. (Chapter 2)
Why it matters: Plaque rupture is a common trigger for coronary clot formation, but plaque erosion and other mechanisms can also cause acute coronary syndromes. Angiographic narrowing alone does not predict which site will cause an event.

Polycystic ovary syndrome (PCOS): a hormonal and metabolic condition that can cause irregular periods and is often associated with insulin resistance. (Chapter 5)
Why it matters: Its cardiovascular importance is that blood pressure, blood sugar, cholesterol, weight, sleep, and other risk factors deserve attention rather than being treated as unrelated problems.

What it does not mean: PCOS does not mean that every woman with the condition will develop heart disease. It is a reason for careful risk-factor review, not a forecast of inevitable events.

See also: *Diabetes / prediabetes; Visceral fat.*

Polygenic risk (polygenic risk score): an estimate that combines many common genetic variants associated with a disease or trait. (Chapter 6)
Why it matters: A score may add information about relative inherited risk, but its usefulness and accuracy can differ among scores, populations, and the decision being considered.
What it does not mean: A high score is not a diagnosis and does not predict exactly what will happen. It should not replace family history, standard risk assessment, or clinical judgment.
See also: *Familial hypercholesterolemia (FH); Lipoprotein(a), or Lp(a).*

Postural orthostatic tachycardia syndrome (POTS): a disorder of orthostatic intolerance in which standing produces symptoms and an excessive, sustained rise in heart rate without the sustained blood-pressure drop that defines orthostatic hypotension. (Chapter 9)
Why it matters: Palpitations and a rapid heart rate have many causes. Diagnosis requires the symptom pattern plus properly measured heart rate and blood pressure while lying and standing or during tilt-table testing.
What it does not mean: A wearable alert for an irregular pulse does not diagnose POTS or atrial fibrillation.
See also: *Atrial fibrillation (AFib); Arrhythmia; Blood pressure (BP).*

Premature menopause: menopause before age 40. (Chapter 5)
Why it matters: Premature menopause is a history that raises cardiovascular risk in current prevention guidance and should prompt careful review of other risks that can be treated.
What it does not mean: It is not a diagnosis of cardiovascular disease and does not determine hormone-therapy decisions by itself.

Primary prevention: lifestyle measures and, when appropriate, medicines used to reduce the chance of a first clinical heart attack, stroke, or other atherosclerotic event in a person without established clinical ASCVD. (Chapter 4)
Why it matters: Risk calculators, calcium scoring, and the intensity of therapy are often approached differently before versus after a clinical event or diagnosis. A younger adult can have low near-term risk while still accumulating long-term exposure.

R

Rate control: a strategy for atrial fibrillation that allows the irregular rhythm to continue while medicines slow the lower chambers so the heart is not racing. (Chapter 9)
Why it matters: Rate control can reduce symptoms and help prevent weakening of the heart from a persistently rapid rate. The target rate is individualized; one number does not fit every patient.
What it does not mean: AFib may still be present, and rate control does not prevent stroke by itself. Anticoagulation is a separate decision based on stroke and bleeding risk.
See also: *Rhythm control; Atrial fibrillation (AFib); Beta blocker; Anticoagulants (including direct oral anticoagulants and warfarin).*

Remodeling (arterial remodeling): the way an artery changes shape as plaque grows, often expanding outward so the inner channel still looks normal on imaging. (Chapter 2)
Why it matters: Outward remodeling can preserve the open inner channel, called the lumen, while plaque accumulates in the wall. Percent narrowing alone can therefore underestimate how much plaque is present. In cardiology, remodeling can also describe changes in the heart's size or shape.
See also: *Plaque; Angiogram (invasive).*

Revascularization: restoring blood flow with a stent (PCI) or bypass surgery (CABG). (Chapter 13)
Why it matters: Revascularization can save heart muscle in selected emergencies, relieve symptoms, and improve outcomes in some forms of high-risk coronary anatomy. Long-term medical care remains important.
See also: *Stent; PCI; CABG.*

Rhythm control: a strategy that tries to restore and maintain a normal heart rhythm with medicine, an electrical reset called cardioversion, a catheter procedure called ablation, or a combination. (Chapter 9)
Why it matters: For selected people with recently diagnosed atrial fibrillation and additional cardiovascular risk, early rhythm control can improve outcomes.
What it does not mean: Rhythm control does not guarantee that AFib will not return, and it does not by itself remove the need for anticoagulation. Rate-control medicine may still be needed.
See also: *Rate control; Atrial fibrillation (AFib); Ablation; Cardioversion; Anticoagulants (including direct oral anticoagulants and warfarin).*

S

SCAD (spontaneous coronary artery dissection): a tear or separation within a coronary artery wall that can squeeze the normal blood channel and cause a heart attack or unstable coronary event. It is not caused by the usual plaque-rupture mechanism. (Chapter 5)
Why it matters: SCAD occurs predominantly in women and often requires a diagnostic and treatment approach different from atherosclerotic coronary disease. Stable patients are frequently managed without an immediate procedure because wires or catheters can sometimes extend the tear.
What it does not mean: SCAD is not the same as aortic dissection, and it cannot be diagnosed from symptoms alone.

Secondary prevention: treatment intended to reduce future events in a person who already has established plaque-related artery disease, such as a prior heart attack, a stroke caused by atherosclerosis, peripheral artery disease causing symptoms, or another established condition.
Why it matters: Starting risk is usually higher after disease is established, so stronger treatment may provide more benefit than it would before disease is known.
What it does not mean: It does not refer only to lifestyle or to a second-line treatment. It is the full prevention strategy after disease is known.

SGLT2 (sodium-glucose cotransporter 2) inhibitors, including empagliflozin and dapagliflozin: medicines used for diabetes, heart failure, and chronic kidney disease indications, with benefits that can extend beyond glucose lowering. (Chapter 14)
Why it matters: For the right patient, an SGLT2 inhibitor can be a central part of treatment. Not everyone with diabetes, heart failure, kidney disease, or coronary plaque needs one.

Silent ischemia (silent myocardial ischemia): objective evidence that heart muscle is not receiving enough blood for its workload even though the person has no angina or related symptoms at that time. (Chapter 8)
Why it matters: The absence of symptoms does not make the finding harmless. Its importance depends on the amount of ischemia, the underlying coronary disease, heart function, and the person's overall risk.
What it does not mean: Silent ischemia is not the same as a silent heart attack. Ischemia means inadequate blood flow; infarction means heart-muscle injury. It also does not mean that every person without symptoms needs routine stress testing.
See also: *Ischemia; Angina; Stress test.*

Stable versus unstable angina: Stable angina follows a familiar, usually exertional pattern. Symptoms that are new, worsening, triggered by less activity than before, or occurring at rest may represent an acute coronary syndrome and require urgent assessment. (Chapter 8)
Why it matters: The distinction is practical and urgent: unstable angina can signal an impending heart attack and needs prompt attention.

Statin: a medication that lowers LDL and ApoB and, importantly, helps stabilize plaque. (Chapter 14)
What it does not mean: An improved LDL is not a reason to stop treatment on your own. The ongoing plan depends on why the statin was prescribed and your current risk.

STEMI (ST-elevation myocardial infarction): an emergency heart-attack pattern on an ECG that usually means a coronary artery has suddenly become severely or completely blocked. Treatment must focus immediately on restoring blood flow.
Why it matters: Minutes matter, but STEMI is not the only life-threatening heart attack. NSTEMI can also be high risk. Treatment is usually urgent PCI when available, but the strategy depends on the clinical situation.

Stenosis: the medical word for a narrowing. It can describe a narrowed artery, heart valve, or another opening in the body.
Why it matters: The location, cause, and degree of narrowing determine what effect it may have. A coronary stenosis may or may not restrict blood flow enough to cause symptoms or justify a procedure.
What it does not mean: Finding a stenosis does not automatically mean that a stent or surgery is needed. Symptoms, blood-flow effects, overall risk, and reasonable alternatives still matter.

Stent: a small metal scaffold placed inside an artery to hold open a specific narrowing. (Chapter 13)
Why it matters: In selected emergencies, especially when a heart attack is caused by a suddenly blocked artery, urgent PCI can save heart muscle and sometimes save a life.
What it does not mean: A stent treats a specific site. It does not remove atherosclerosis elsewhere or replace medicines and risk-factor treatment when those are indicated.
See also: *Revascularization; PCI; CABG.*

Stress test: a test that looks for signs that heart muscle is not receiving enough blood during exercise or medication-induced stress; some forms also measure exercise capacity. (Chapter 12)
What it does not mean: A normal result means no evidence of reduced heart-muscle blood flow was detected under the conditions tested. It does not show all plaque, predict which plaque may break open, or rule out every problem in the heart's smallest vessels.

Stroke: brain injury caused by interrupted blood flow (ischemic stroke) or bleeding in or around the brain (hemorrhagic stroke).
Why it matters: Sudden facial drooping, one-sided weakness or numbness, trouble speaking or understanding speech, vision loss, severe imbalance, or a sudden severe headache requires emergency care; call 911.
What it does not mean: Not every stroke is caused by atherosclerosis or atrial fibrillation.
See also: *ASCVD; Atrial fibrillation (AFib); Anticoagulants.*

T

Takotsubo syndrome: a temporary weakening of the heart muscle that can follow intense physical or emotional stress and can resemble a heart attack. (Chapters 5 and 15)
Why it matters: Chest pain, ECG changes, and heart-muscle injury require urgent evaluation because a plaque-related heart attack and other emergencies must be ruled out.

Troponin: a protein released into the blood when heart muscle is injured. (Chapter 12)
Why it matters: Repeat troponin measurements are interpreted with symptoms, ECG findings, imaging, and the time symptoms began. A high value is not automatically a heart attack, and one early normal value may not be enough to rule one out.

Type 1 and Type 2 myocardial infarction: A Type 1 heart attack usually occurs when plaque breaks open or erodes and a new clot sharply reduces coronary blood flow. A Type 2 heart attack occurs when the heart needs more oxygen than the blood can supply because of another major strain, without a new plaque-related clot. The formal classification also includes Types 3, 4, and 5 for specific death- and procedure-related settings; this book focuses on Types 1 and 2.
Why it matters: Severe anemia, very low blood oxygen, sepsis, a sustained rapid heart rhythm, very high blood pressure, or very low blood pressure can contribute to a Type 2 heart attack. Evaluation and treatment focus on the cause as well as underlying coronary risk.
What it does not mean: Type 2 does not mean unimportant, and a high troponin alone does not establish either type. A heart attack requires evidence of a recent lack of blood flow to heart muscle; heart-muscle injury from another cause is a different diagnosis.

V

Variant of uncertain significance (VUS): a genetic finding for which the evidence is not yet settled as to whether the variant causes or contributes to disease. (Chapter 6)
Why it matters: Laboratories generally classify variants as pathogenic, likely pathogenic, uncertain, likely benign, or benign. A VUS should not, by itself, diagnose a condition, change treatment, or be used for predictive testing of relatives as though it were definitive. Its classification can change as evidence grows.
What it does not mean: A VUS is not the same as a pathogenic or likely pathogenic result. Keep a copy of the complete report and ask the genetics team or laboratory how updated interpretations are communicated.
See also: *Familial hypercholesterolemia (FH); Polygenic risk (polygenic risk score); Cascade screening.*

Visceral fat: fat stored within the abdominal cavity around internal organs. (Chapter 4)
Why it matters: More visceral fat is associated with insulin resistance, fatty liver disease, abnormal cholesterol or triglycerides, and a higher risk of diabetes and cardiovascular disease.
What it does not mean: Body mass index (BMI) does not directly measure visceral fat or define cardiovascular health. Waist measurement, laboratory values, blood pressure, fitness, and the full clinical picture add context.

Vulnerable plaque: an informal term for plaque with features associated with a higher risk of disruption, such as a thin cap, large lipid core, or substantial plaque burden. (Chapter 2)
Why it matters: Features associated with plaque vulnerability can add information beyond percent narrowing, but no feature predicts an individual event with certainty.

Numbers

90-Day Plan: this book's three-month planning framework: safety and stabilization, building capacity, and review and adjustment. The emphases overlap rather than beginning and ending on exact dates. (Chapter 16)
Why it matters: Ninety days is a practical review period, not a biological deadline. The plan should be adapted to diagnoses, recovery, ability, resources, and clinician guidance.

Selected References and Key Studies

This representative selection includes major trials, cohort studies, reviews, and scientific statements relevant to the book. The evidence was reviewed through July 2026. It is a starting point rather than a systematic review, and current guidelines should be consulted for clinical decisions.

Plaque Biology, Endothelial Dysfunction & Flow

These studies show that risk reflects total plaque burden and plaque features as well as the degree of narrowing. No plaque feature predicts an individual event with certainty.

- INTERHEART Study. Yusuf S, Hawken S, Ôunpuu S, et al. Effect of potentially modifiable risk factors associated with myocardial infarction in 52 countries. Lancet. 2004;364:937–952.
- PROSPECT Trial. Stone GW, Maehara A, Lansky AJ, et al. A prospective natural-history study of coronary atherosclerosis. N Engl J Med. 2011;364:226–235.
- CONFIRM Registry. Min JK, Dunning A, Lin FY, et al. Age- and sex-related differences in mortality risk by CCTA findings. J Am Coll Cardiol. 2011;58:849–860.
- MESA Study. Detrano R, Guerci AD, Carr JJ, et al. Coronary calcium as a predictor of events across diverse populations. N Engl J Med. 2008;358:1336–1345.

- ICONIC Study. Chang HJ, Lin FY, Lee SE, et al. Coronary atherosclerotic precursors of acute coronary syndromes. J Am Coll Cardiol. 2018;71:2511–2522. doi:10.1016/j.jacc.2018.02.079.
- Zaman T, Agarwal S, Anabtawi AG, et al. Angiographic lesion severity and subsequent myocardial infarction. Am J Cardiol. 2012;110:167–172. doi:10.1016/j.amjcard.2012.03.008.

Inflammation & Residual Risk

These trials helped establish inflammation as one pathway in atherosclerosis. JUPITER tested statin therapy in selected patients with elevated hs-CRP; CANTOS tested targeted anti-inflammatory therapy after myocardial infarction.

- JUPITER Trial. Ridker PM, Danielson E, Fonseca FAH, et al. Rosuvastatin to prevent vascular events in men and women with elevated C-reactive protein. N Engl J Med. 2008;359:2195–2207.
- CANTOS Trial. Ridker PM, Everett BM, Thuren T, et al. Antiinflammatory therapy with canakinumab for atherosclerotic disease. N Engl J Med. 2017;377:1119–1131.

Blood Pressure, Vascular Injury & Protection

These trials support careful blood-pressure control and risk-reducing therapy in appropriately selected high-risk patients.

- SPRINT Trial. SPRINT Research Group. Intensive versus standard blood-pressure control. N Engl J Med. 2015;373:2103–2116.
- HOPE Trial. Yusuf S, Sleight P, Pogue J, et al. ACE inhibition and cardiovascular outcomes in high-risk patients. N Engl J Med. 2000;342:145–153.

Lipids, ApoB, Lp(a) & Plaque Stabilization

These studies show that lowering ApoB-containing particles reduces cardiovascular events and that Lp(a) is a largely inherited, measurable risk factor.

- Heart Protection Study. Cholesterol lowering in high-risk individuals. Lancet. 2002;360:7–22.
- PROVE-IT TIMI-22. Cannon CP, Braunwald E, McCabe CH, et al. Intensive vs moderate statin therapy after acute coronary syndrome. N Engl J Med. 2004;350:1495–1504.
- FOURIER Trial. Sabatine MS, Giugliano RP, Keech AC, et al. Evolocumab and outcomes in cardiovascular disease. N Engl J Med. 2017;376:1713–1722.
- ODYSSEY OUTCOMES. Schwartz GG, Steg PG, Szarek M, et al. Alirocumab after acute coronary syndrome. N Engl J Med. 2018;379:2097–2107.
- Lipoprotein(a) Measurement. Marcovina SM, Shapiro MD. Measurement of lipoprotein(a): a once-in-a-lifetime opportunity. J Am Coll Cardiol. 2022;79:629–631.
- NLA Lp(a) Scientific Statement (Focused Update). Koschinsky ML, Bajaj A, Boffa MB, et al. A focused update to the 2019 National Lipid Association statement on use of lipoprotein(a) in clinical practice. J Clin Lipidol. 2024;18:e308–e319.
- 2026 Dyslipidemia Guideline. Blumenthal RS, Morris PB, Gaudino M, et al. 2026 ACC/AHA/AACVPR/ABC/ACPM/ADA/AGS/APhA/ASPC/NLA/PCNA Guideline on the Management of Dyslipidemia: A Report of the American College of Cardiology/American Heart Association Joint Committee on Clinical Practice Guidelines. J Am Coll Cardiol. 2026;87(19):2624–2757. doi:10.1016/j.jacc.2025.11.016. (Recommends measuring Lp(a) at least once in every adult and introduces risk-based LDL-C treatment goals.)

- CLEAR Outcomes Trial. Nissen SE, Lincoff AM, Brennan D, et al. Bempedoic acid in statin-intolerant patients. N Engl J Med. 2023;388:1353–1364.

Diabetes, Metabolic Health & Incretin Therapies

These trials show that selected diabetes and weight-management medicines improve cardiovascular outcomes in defined patient groups. The drugs and populations are not interchangeable.

- UKPDS 33 & Follow-Up. Intensive glucose control and long-term outcomes. Lancet. 1998;352:837–853; N Engl J Med. 2008;359:1577–1589.
- EMPA-REG OUTCOME. Zinman B, Wanner C, Lachin JM, et al. Empagliflozin and cardiovascular mortality. N Engl J Med. 2015;373:2117–2128.
- SELECT Trial. Lincoff AM, Brown-Frandsen K, Colhoun HM, et al. Semaglutide and cardiovascular outcomes in overweight or obesity without diabetes. N Engl J Med. 2023;389:2221–2232.
- SURPASS-CVOT. Nicholls SJ, Pavo I, Bhatt DL, et al. Cardiovascular outcomes with tirzepatide versus dulaglutide in type 2 diabetes. N Engl J Med. 2025;393(24):2409–2420. doi:10.1056/NEJMoa2505928.

Women's Cardiovascular Disease & Microvascular Flow

These studies and statements address ischemia without obstructive disease, menopause, adverse pregnancy outcomes, and important nonatherosclerotic causes of acute cardiac events in women.

- WISE Study. Bairey Merz CN, Shaw LJ, Reis SE, et al. Gender differences in ischemic heart disease. J Am Coll Cardiol. 2006;47(3 Suppl):S21–S29.

- Menopause Transition and Cardiovascular Risk. El Khoudary SR, Aggarwal B, Beckie TM, et al. A scientific statement from the American Heart Association. Circulation. 2020;142:e506–e532. doi:10.1161/CIR.0000000000000912.
- Adverse Pregnancy Outcomes and Cardiovascular Risk. Parikh NI, Gonzalez JM, Anderson CAM, et al. A scientific statement from the American Heart Association. Circulation. 2021;143:e902–e916. doi:10.1161/CIR.0000000000000961.
- Women's Health Initiative Timing Analysis. Rossouw JE, Prentice RL, Manson JE, et al. Hormone therapy and cardiovascular risk by age and years since menopause. JAMA. 2007;297:1465–1477.
- Lp(a) in Pregnancy. Makvandi S, Karimi L, Larki M, et al. Lipoprotein(a) in pregnancy: a systematic review and meta-analysis. Prog Cardiovasc Dis. 2025;92:161–179. doi:10.1016/j.pcad.2025.07.012.
- Coronary Microvascular Dysfunction. Camici PG, Crea F. Coronary microvascular dysfunction. N Engl J Med. 2007;356:830–840.
- CorMicA Trial. Ford TJ, Stanley B, Good R, et al. Stratified medical therapy using invasive coronary function testing in angina. J Am Coll Cardiol. 2018;72:2841–2855.
- Microvascular Disease Review. Taqueti VR, Di Carli MF. Coronary microvascular disease: pathogenic mechanisms and therapeutic options. J Am Coll Cardiol. 2018;72:2625–2641.
- Vasospastic Angina Criteria. Beltrame JF, Crea F, Kaski JC, et al. International standardization of diagnostic criteria for vasospastic angina. Eur Heart J. 2017;38:2565–2568.
- Spontaneous Coronary Artery Dissection. Hayes SN, Kim ESH, Saw J, et al. A scientific statement from the American Heart Association. Circulation. 2018;137:e523–e557. doi:10.1161/CIR.0000000000000564.

- MINOCA Scientific Statement. Tamis-Holland JE, Jneid H, Reynolds HR, et al. Contemporary diagnosis and management of myocardial infarction in the absence of obstructive coronary artery disease. Circulation. 2019;139:e891–e908. doi:10.1161/CIR.0000000000000670.

Stents, Revascularization & Medical Therapy

These trials clarify the different roles of urgent revascularization, symptom-relieving PCI, physiology-guided treatment, and medical therapy in acute and stable coronary disease.

- COURAGE Trial. Boden WE, O'Rourke RA, Teo KK, et al. PCI versus optimal medical therapy in stable coronary disease. N Engl J Med. 2007;356:1503–1516.
- ISCHEMIA Trial. Maron DJ, Hochman JS, Reynolds HR, et al. Initial invasive or conservative strategy for stable coronary disease. N Engl J Med. 2020;382:1395–1407.
- FAME Trial. Tonino PAL, De Bruyne B, Pijls NHJ, et al. Fractional flow reserve versus angiography for guiding PCI. N Engl J Med. 2009;360:213–224.
- FAME 2 Trial. De Bruyne B, Pijls NHJ, Kalesan B, et al. Fractional flow reserve-guided PCI versus medical therapy in stable coronary disease. N Engl J Med. 2012;367:991–1001.
- FAME 2 Five-Year Follow-Up. Xaplanteris P, Fournier S, Pijls NHJ, et al. Five-year outcomes with PCI guided by fractional flow reserve. N Engl J Med. 2018;379(3):250–259. doi:10.1056/NEJMoa1803538.
- ORBITA Trial. Al-Lamee R, Thompson D, Dehbi HM, et al. Percutaneous coronary intervention in stable angina: a double-blind, randomized, sham-controlled trial. Lancet. 2018;391:31–40.
- PREVENT Trial. Park S-J, Ahn J-M, Kang D-Y, et al. Preventive PCI versus optimal medical therapy for selected vulnerable plaques. Lancet. 2024;403:1753–1765.

- REDUCE-AMI Trial. Yndigegn T, Lindahl B, Mars K, et al. Beta-blockers after myocardial infarction and preserved ejection fraction. N Engl J Med. 2024;390:1372–1381.
- REBOOT-CNIC Trial. Ibanez B, Latini R, Rossello X, et al. Beta-blockers after myocardial infarction without reduced ejection fraction. N Engl J Med. 2025;393(19):1889–1900. doi:10.1056/NEJMoa2504735.
- Contemporary Beta-Blocker Evidence. Kristensen AMD, Rossello X, Atar D, et al. Beta-blockers after myocardial infarction with normal ejection fraction. N Engl J Med. 2026;394(6):540–550. doi:10.1056/NEJMoa2512686.

Genetics and Inherited Risk

These studies describe the genetic architecture of coronary disease and show how inherited susceptibility interacts with lifestyle.

- Genetic Risk and Lifestyle. Khera AV, Emdin CA, Drake I, et al. Genetic risk, adherence to a healthy lifestyle, and coronary disease. N Engl J Med. 2016;375:2349–2358.
- CARDIoGRAMplusC4D Consortium. Nikpay M, Goel A, Won HH, et al. A comprehensive genome-wide association meta-analysis of coronary artery disease. Nat Genet. 2015;47:1121–1130.
- 9p21 Locus and Coronary Disease. McPherson R, Pertsemlidis A, Kavaslar N, et al. Science. 2007;316:1488–1491.
- 9p21 Locus and Myocardial Infarction. Helgadottir A, Thorleifsson G, Manolescu A, et al. Science. 2007;316:1491–1493.
- Genome-Wide Analysis of CAD. Samani NJ, Erdmann J, Hall AS, et al. N Engl J Med. 2007;357:443–453.

Emerging Tests and Treatments

These investigations cover evolving imaging markers, Lp(a)-lowering drugs, and artificial intelligence in cardiovascular care. They are a current snapshot; several tools and outcome questions remain investigational.

- CRISP-CT Study. Oikonomou EK, Marwan M, Desai MY, et al. Noninvasive detection of coronary inflammation using CT and prediction of residual risk. Lancet. 2018;392:929–939.
- ORFAN Study. Chan K, Wahome E, Tsiachristas A, et al. Inflammatory risk and cardiovascular events without obstructive coronary disease. Lancet. 2024;403:2606–2618.
- Pelacarsen Phase 2. Tsimikas S, Karwatowska-Prokopczuk E, Gouni-Berthold I, et al. Lipoprotein(a) reduction in persons with cardiovascular disease. N Engl J Med. 2020;382:244–255.
- Olpasiran OCEAN(a)-DOSE. O'Donoghue ML, Rosenson RS, Gencer B, et al. Small interfering RNA to reduce lipoprotein(a). N Engl J Med. 2022;387:1855–1864.
- Lp(a) Outcomes Trials. Lp(a)HORIZON (NCT04023552) and OCEAN(a)-Outcomes (NCT05581303). Outcomes evidence remains under study at the time of publication.
- Artificial Intelligence in Cardiovascular Medicine. Lüscher TF, Wenzl FA, D'Ascenzo F, Friedman PA, Antoniades C. Eur Heart J. 2024;45:4291–4304.

Current Clinical Practice Guidelines

These are the major guidelines used for the book's recommendations on blood pressure, coronary disease, chest pain, stents and bypass surgery, heart failure, and the connected care of the heart, kidneys, and metabolism.

- High Blood Pressure Guideline. Jones DW, Ferdinand KC, Taler SJ, et al. 2025 AHA/ACC/AANP/AAPA/ABC/ACCP/ACPM/AGS/AMA/ASPC/NMA/PCNA/SGIM Guideline for the Prevention, Detection, Evaluation and Management of High Blood Pressure in Adults: A Report of the American College of Cardiology/American Heart Association Joint Committee on Clinical Practice Guidelines. Circulation. 2025;152(11):e114–e218. doi:10.1161/CIR.0000000000001356.
- Acute Coronary Syndromes Guideline. Rao SV, O'Donoghue ML, Ruel M, et al. 2025 ACC/AHA/ACEP/NAEMSP/SCAI Guideline for the Management of Patients With Acute Coronary Syndromes: A Report of the American College of Cardiology/American Heart Association Joint Committee on Clinical Practice Guidelines. Circulation. 2025;151(13):e771–e862. doi:10.1161/CIR.0000000000001309.
- Chronic Coronary Disease Guideline. Virani SS, Newby LK, Arnold SV, et al. 2023 AHA/ACC/ACCP/ASPC/NLA/PCNA Guideline for the Management of Patients With Chronic Coronary Disease. Circulation. 2023;148:e9–e119. doi:10.1161/CIR.0000000000001168.
- Heart Failure Guideline. Heidenreich PA, Bozkurt B, Aguilar D, et al. 2022 AHA/ACC/HFSA Guideline for the Management of Heart Failure. Circulation. 2022;145:e895–e1032. doi:10.1161/CIR.0000000000001063.
- Walsh MN, Kober L, Sliwa K, et al. AHA/ACC/ESC/WHF Expert Consensus Document: Second Universal Definition of Heart Failure (2026). Circulation. Published online June 29, 2026. doi:10.1161/CIR.0000000000001455.
- Chest Pain Guideline. Gulati M, Levy PD, Mukherjee D, et al. 2021 AHA/ACC/ASE/CHEST/SAEM/SCCT/SCMR Guideline for the Evaluation and Diagnosis of Chest Pain. Circulation. 2021;144:e368–e454. doi:10.1161/CIR.0000000000001029.

- Coronary Revascularization Guideline. Lawton JS, Tamis-Holland JE, Bangalore S, et al. 2021 ACC/AHA/SCAI Guideline for Coronary Artery Revascularization. Circulation. 2022;145:e18–e114. doi:10.1161/CIR.0000000000001038.
- Cardiovascular-Kidney-Metabolic Syndrome Guideline. Ndumele CE, Rodriguez F, Dixon DL, et al. 2026 AHA/ACC/ADA/ASN Guideline for the Prevention, Detection, Evaluation, and Management of Cardiovascular-Kidney-Metabolic Syndrome: A Report of the American College of Cardiology/American Heart Association Joint Committee on Clinical Practice Guidelines. Circulation. Published online June 9, 2026. doi:10.1161/CIR.0000000000001453.

Rhythm and Atrial Fibrillation

These sources support AFib diagnosis, stroke prevention, wearable alerts, early rhythm control, and decisions about brief episodes detected by implanted cardiac devices.

- Atrial Fibrillation Guideline. Joglar JA, Chung MK, Armbruster AL, et al. 2023 ACC/AHA/ACCP/HRS Guideline for the Diagnosis and Management of Atrial Fibrillation. Circulation. 2024;149:e1–e156. doi:10.1161/CIR.0000000000001193.
- Early Rhythm Control (EAST-AFNET 4). Kirchhof P, Camm AJ, Goette A, et al. Early rhythm-control therapy in patients with atrial fibrillation. N Engl J Med. 2020;383:1305–1316. doi:10.1056/NEJMoa2019422.
- Device-Detected AFib (ARTESiA). Healey JS, Lopes RD, Granger CB, et al. Apixaban for stroke prevention in subclinical atrial fibrillation. N Engl J Med. 2024;390:107–117. doi:10.1056/NEJMoa2310234.

- Atrial High-Rate Episodes (NOAH-AFNET 6). Kirchhof P, Toennis T, Goette A, et al. Anticoagulation with edoxaban in patients with atrial high-rate episodes. N Engl J Med. 2023;389:1167–1179. doi:10.1056/NEJMoa2303062.
- ALONE-AF Trial. Kim D, Shim J, Choi E-K, et al. Long-term anticoagulation discontinuation after catheter ablation for atrial fibrillation. JAMA. 2025;334(14):1246–1254. doi:10.1001/jama.2025.14679.
- OCEAN Trial. Verma A, Birnie D, Jiang C, et al. Antithrombotic therapy after successful catheter ablation for atrial fibrillation. N Engl J Med. 2026;394(4):323–332. doi:10.1056/NEJMoa2509688.
- Apple Heart Study. Perez MV, Mahaffey KW, Hedlin H, et al. Large-scale assessment of a smartwatch to identify atrial fibrillation. N Engl J Med. 2019;381:1909–1917. doi:10.1056/NEJMoa1901183.

Sleep and Obstructive Sleep Apnea

These sources support the discussion of cardiovascular associations, diagnostic evaluation, CPAP benefits, and the limits of cardiovascular-event claims.

- Sleep-Disordered Breathing and Hypertension. Peppard PE, Young T, Palta M, Skatrud J. N Engl J Med. 2000;342:1378–1384.
- Obstructive Sleep Apnea and Outcomes. Marin JM, Carrizo SJ, Vicente E, Agustí AGN. Lancet. 2005;365:1046–1053.
- Obstructive Sleep Apnea and Cardiovascular Disease. Yeghiazarians Y, Jneid H, Tietjens JR, et al. Circulation. 2021;144:e56–e67. doi:10.1161/CIR.0000000000000988.
- CPAP and Cardiovascular Events (SAVE). McEvoy RD, Antic NA, Heeley E, et al. N Engl J Med. 2016;375:919–931. doi:10.1056/NEJMoa1606599.

- Adult OSA Diagnostic Testing Guideline. Kapur VK, Auckley DH, Chowdhuri S, et al. Clinical practice guideline for diagnostic testing for adult obstructive sleep apnea. J Clin Sleep Med. 2017;13(3):479–504. doi:10.5664/jcsm.6506.
- SURMOUNT-OSA. Malhotra A, Grunstein RR, Fietze I, et al. Tirzepatide for the treatment of obstructive sleep apnea and obesity. N Engl J Med. 2024;391:1193–1205. doi:10.1056/NEJMoa2404881.

Recovery, Psychological Health, and Takotsubo

These sources support the discussion of psychological recovery, antidepressant safety, cardiac rehabilitation, and Takotsubo syndrome.

- Cardiac Rehabilitation. Dibben G, Faulkner J, Oldridge N, et al. Exercise-based cardiac rehabilitation for coronary heart disease. Cochrane Database Syst Rev. 2021;11:CD001800.
- Bereavement and Acute MI Risk. Mostofsky E, Maclure M, Sherwood JB, et al. Circulation. 2012;125:491–496.
- Post-Myocardial Infarction Psychological Distress. Levine GN, Carney RM, Cohen BE, et al. Post-myocardial infarction psychological distress: a scientific statement from the American Heart Association. Circulation. 2025;152(16):e298–e310. doi:10.1161/CIR.0000000000001381.
- SADHART. Glassman AH, O'Connor CM, Califf RM, et al. Sertraline treatment of major depression in patients with acute myocardial infarction or unstable angina. JAMA. 2002;288:701–709. doi:10.1001/jama.288.6.701.
- Contemporary Cardiac Rehabilitation (CaReMATCH). Stens NA, Buckley BJR, Dibben GO, et al. Exercise-based cardiac rehabilitation for coronary heart disease: the CaReMATCH individual participant data meta-analysis. Eur J Prev Cardiol. 2026;33(6):841–853. doi:10.1093/eurjpc/zwaf629.

- Takotsubo Syndrome Consensus, Part II. Ghadri JR, Wittstein IS, Prasad A, et al. Eur Heart J. 2018;39:2047–2062. doi:10.1093/eurheartj/ehy077.
- Core Components of Cardiac Rehabilitation. Brown TM, Pack QR, Aberegg E, et al. Core components of cardiac rehabilitation programs: 2024 update: a scientific statement from the American Heart Association and the American Association of Cardiovascular and Pulmonary Rehabilitation. Circulation. 2024;150(18):e328-e347. doi:10.1161/CIR.0000000000001289.

Diet, Physical Activity, and Tobacco Treatment

- AHA Dietary Guidance. Lichtenstein AH, Appel LJ, Vadiveloo M, et al. 2021 dietary guidance to improve cardiovascular health: a scientific statement from the American Heart Association. Circulation. 2021;144(23):e472-e487. doi:10.1161/CIR.0000000000001031.
- PREDIMED, Corrected Report. Estruch R, Ros E, Salas-Salvadó J, et al. Primary prevention of cardiovascular disease with a Mediterranean diet supplemented with extra-virgin olive oil or nuts. N Engl J Med. 2018;378(25):e34. doi:10.1056/NEJMoa1800389.
- Physical Activity Guidelines. U.S. Department of Health and Human Services. Physical Activity Guidelines for Americans. 2nd ed. Washington, DC: U.S. Department of Health and Human Services; 2018.
- Smoking Cessation. U.S. Department of Health and Human Services. Smoking Cessation: A Report of the Surgeon General. Atlanta, GA: U.S. Department of Health and Human Services, Centers for Disease Control and Prevention, National Center for Chronic Disease Prevention and Health Promotion, Office on Smoking and Health; 2020.

Supplements and Prescription Omega-3 Therapy

- REDUCE-IT. Bhatt DL, Steg PG, Miller M, et al. Cardiovascular risk reduction with icosapent ethyl for hypertriglyceridemia. N Engl J Med. 2019;380(1):11–22. doi:10.1056/NEJMoa1812792.
- STRENGTH. Nicholls SJ, Lincoff AM, Garcia M, et al. Effect of high-dose omega-3 fatty acids vs corn oil on major adverse cardiovascular events in patients at high cardiovascular risk: the STRENGTH randomized clinical trial. JAMA. 2020;324(22):2268–2280. doi:10.1001/jama.2020.22258.
- HPS2-THRIVE. HPS2-THRIVE Collaborative Group. Effects of extended-release niacin with laropiprant in high-risk patients. N Engl J Med. 2014;371(3):203–212. doi:10.1056/NEJMoa1300955.
- AIM-HIGH. AIM-HIGH Investigators. Niacin in patients with low HDL cholesterol levels receiving intensive statin therapy. N Engl J Med. 2011;365(24):2255–2267. doi:10.1056/NEJMoa1107579.
- VITAL. Manson JE, Cook NR, Lee IM, et al. Vitamin D supplements and prevention of cancer and cardiovascular disease. N Engl J Med. 2019;380(1):33–44. doi:10.1056/NEJMoa1809944.
- Red Yeast Rice Safety. National Center for Complementary and Integrative Health. Red yeast rice: what you need to know. Updated November 2022. Accessed July 10, 2026. https://www.nccih.nih.gov/health/red-yeast-rice.

www.ingramcontent.com/pod-product-compliance
Lightning Source LLC
LaVergne TN
LVHW051921051126
851857LV00021B/2095